NeverSeconds

NeverSeconds

Martha Payne and David Payne

"NeverSeconds: The Incredible Story of Martha Payne"
Dave Payne & Martha Payne

First Published 2012
Published by Cargo Publishing
SC376700
ISBN: 978-1908885166
Bic Code: BT Biography: True Stories

Cover design and typesetting by Freight Design

Cover photography by Chris Watt

Printed and bound by Bell and Bain, Glasgow

For all the children receiving Mary's Meals.

May your number continue to grow.

Introduction

I first met Martha Payne when I set up a meeting to discuss the state of school meals and food education. I'd been at a conference three months before and promised to restart a proper discussion about improving school meals for kids across the board.

Little did I know, but a 9-year-old girl from Lochgilphead had a similar idea. Like me, she thought the food served in school wasn't really good enough, and like me, she wondered what to do about it. Where I decided to set up a meeting with politicians, food providers and the like, she began writing a blog, NeverSeconds, starting with the simple act of taking a daily photo of her lunch and rating the meals out of 10.

I'm a parent with a daughter the same age as Martha and what I feed my kids matters hugely to me. Martha's pictures struck such a chord with me – and thousands of other parents, who saw the images and thought: 'Is that really what my kids are eating at school?'

So I invited her along to the meeting with her Dad to judge the 'school' lunches made by everyone at the meeting to a strict budget of £1.05 – and, like on her blog, give everyone a mark out of 10.

Martha's amazing story that spun from the day she took the first picture of a paltry bit of pizza and a few desultory scraps of sweetcorn, to the day she came to my Cook School and a tabloid snap caused a giant furore, shows us many things. First, everyone can change the world – not only has Martha brought attention to what we feed our kids, but she's also managed to raise over £120,000 for children who have virtually nothing to eat in Africa. Her chosen charity, Mary's Meals, provides hungry

African children with daily hot meals at school – thereby also encouraging them to come and be educated.

Martha's story also highlights the fact that we in the rich West don't always feed our children what's best for them. One of the most interesting parts of Martha's blog is the images people from all over the world send in of their lunches. From Japan, Korea, India, China and elsewhere, meals in countries far poorer than the UK outshine ours in terms of quality, appearance, and nutritional value by a mile.

I've now met Martha a few times, and what I really like about her is that she's totally genuine. She's not precocious. She's just a straight-talking, very honest 9-year-old girl, with a great family behind her, who tells it like it is.

Good on ya Martha. You've already achieved great things. Don't forget to keep stirring that porridge.

Nick Nairn

The Seed

It was something my dad had done for me when I was Martha's age. Holding a plate low over a candle until a thin layer of soot formed as the flame struggled for air. It was Martha's class open evening all about the Titanic and she had chosen that we would all be members of the 'black gang', the stokers that fuelled the boilers with coal. So in our finest work clothes we were applying the finishing touches.

The plate was getting warm as I moved it slowly over the candle and the greasy black makeup was easily wiped in dramatic smears across our faces. Martha was the last to go and was giggling at the sight of her Mum, Rebecca, who moments before had burled into the house from her job as a local General Practitioner in her smart work outfit only to reappear minutes later in boots and a jumper two sizes too big. The dark lines I'd drawn on her face exaggerated her features and made her look very tired. Being tired was something she often was, as a GP and a mum. It was luck that she wasn't on call that night, so she could enjoy dressing up with the rest of us without fear that at any moment she may have to dash to the hospital to appear over a casualty with her new look.

Martha's older brother, Joe, needed less help to look ragged. Holes in his trouser knees and trainers were the norm and he sported the traditionally unkempt hair of an eleven-year-old boy. He was champing at the bit, edging to the door with promises of beating us to the school on his bike and with a nod from Mum he grabbed his fluorescent vest and was gone. I had no idea what passersby would make of him with soot on his face and hands but with Lochgilphead being a small town most folk would know there was an event at the school.

Polly, Martha's seven-year-old little sister, was frustrated not to have been first in the queue for soot but typically it had taken her three changes of outfit before she was confident it was the best costume she could muster. Four changes of shoes and she had slipped behind Joe for sooting up. I was trying to explain to her why the soot formed as I moved the plate so low that the candle spluttered and came close to dying. Polly wasn't interested in my explanation of the combustion triangle, fuel, air and heat, for a clean burn. She was more interested to see if I could produce a colour other than black.

"I quite like blue Dad," was her request and my failure to produce eye makeup in duck blue was written all over her face as she scrumpled it up. Polly, like Martha, had one of those cheeky happy faces that go from creased upset to broad smile in an instant and as she slipped her glasses back on to see herself in the mirror she did just that. Pleased with her transformation she grabbed an apple and disappeared.

Martha had been telling us all about the Titanic for a couple of weeks. We knew the number of boilers, the captain's name, the way crew and passengers were segregated and even the menus on offer to the first class passengers. Out of all the classes of passenger and all the staff roles she had been most captivated by the 'black gang'. The dirtiest members of the crew that slogged away in the depths of the ship and yet on whose work the whole operation of the ship hinged. I was glad. Trying to dress as a first class passenger would have been beyond my smallholder's wardrobe. In fact I had very few smart clothes at all. Hanging in my space there were a few shirts, mainly checked, and my climbing harness and caving suit. It had been years, more than a decade in fact, since either were used but it wasn't until we moved to our smallholding that I stopped introducing myself as an ex mountaineering instructor and househusband. Even that was an exaggeration. I'd spent many happy years working with young people, some troubled and some disabled, introducing them to climbing, kayaking and caving. Whilst I had qualifications that would allow me to label myself a professional mountaineer the truth was I preferred to be on the hills and cliffs with youngsters whose enthusiasm could be supported rather than grizzled climbers who wished

to discuss the relative merits of an alpine butterfly over a figure of 16 knot. The standard line I developed over those early years of being a househusband was to say:

"When Rebecca and I found out we were expecting we got our payslips out and compared them. I am not sure whether I won or lost but I have been at home ever since!"

Those early years surrounded at playgroups by mums were a challenge. An incident when I was invited to take Joe, who was only four months old at the time, to a colleague of Rebecca's for a play date with two other mums was a defining moment. The kids were rolling on the floor and it became clear, as one of the mums bent over, that she was wearing a pair of narrow G-string knickers. Feeling slightly awkward I picked Joe up from my knee and put him down amongst the toys with the words, "There you go Joe. Go and join the thong."

Whilst my brain was screaming, 'I meant throng, I meant throng,' my attempts to explain only dug me deeper into the hole I had made myself. I left red faced, awkward, embarrassed and never to be invited again. So when we moved to Lochgilphead it took an incredible effort to join the playgroups and Rebecca had to cajole me along. She met many mums through the surgery and soon I became very used to being asked if I was the new doctor's husband. In fact it soon felt like my latest job title.

Martha had been waiting quietly, filling in the boarding pass she had brought home from school. It was typical of her class teacher, Mr Maddox, to use every opportunity to draw the children and families into the story. It was teaching at its best. Martha was learning about social change, engineering and history, and she was doing it through drama, model building and writing, but more than that she was having fun. Completely engaged in filling out her boarding pass Martha was showing her determination to do things properly.

As parents across the world have done before me, I often wished for an off switch on my children; on some a switch for noise, on others a switch for excitement, but for Martha a switch for determination would have been very useful. From the boarding pass that had to be in the flowery script of an Edwardian clerk to the battles over bedtime, her will could be both the hardest thing to cope with and her strongest asset. I wanted all

my children to grow strong and happy, and to be able to take on and enjoy the world. Streaking soot diagonally from her ear to the corner of her mouth Martha was gabbling with excitement. Once finished, she took off to the car and we followed. A rag tag family dressed in rags and covered in soot, off to explore a classroom converted into the Titanic. As the ship set off on its journey we were unwittingly setting off a chain of events that would take us all on the journey of a lifetime.

Not everyone in our house was a morning person and the day after the Titanic sank for the second time was no exception. The classroom walls had been covered in the work the children had done on the topic. There were inventories, life stories of the captain and crew, details of the radio operators and how the ship was navigated. Across three tables was a model in cross section of the ship, which stood as a testament to the hard work of the class. The evening ended the same way as it did in April 1912 with us all squeezing into a small space; singing with the band as we watched the cold Atlantic waters flooding in and all finally was lost. No surprise then that the morning after wasn't the smoothest as tiredness gave way to a new day.

The morning routine in our house had developed to soothe the pain of getting up whilst allowing me to get around the important jobs on the smallholding. A smallholding had been a dream for many years. We grew vegetables and kept hens at our old small cottage but really lacked the space to do much more. Many an evening I had sketched out plans for an imaginary five acres with dotted lines for fences, triangles for gates and crosses for apple trees. It wasn't until 2007 that the perfect place came onto the market and we were able to make a reality from our plans. I still wasn't bringing any money in but I placed good food on the table every day instead. All those evenings of triangles and crosses paid off and soon we had divided our six acres of grazing into pig paddocks, two meadows and an orchard. Surrounded by woods and alongside the Crinan Canal we had the space to produce enough for us, and a surplus to share.

Starting off as a smallholder we were constantly faced with challenges that seemed to need a special tool or specialist knowledge, and time after time the support of friends was the

difference between success and spectacular failure. The culture of helping each other was deep seated and respected. It was the norm here and some of the most difficult chats I had with friends were not because I was asking too much of them but that I was asking too little. Concerned I had nothing to offer my farming friends in return they patiently pointed out to me that I did not need to help them but just help somebody. So as I set off on my morning rounds to check on the stock, the lamb gang bouncing around the ewes was as much a testament to the kindness of the farmer who had lent us a good ram and our cycling shepherd friend who had helped get the ewes in top condition, than to having six acres of grass to keep them on. The pigs greeted me with squeals and a new ambush tactic. Most commonly the three Tamworths would divide into two forces and a pair would focus on the feed bucket whilst the loan ace would wheel behind and go for the wellies.

Today was different. Instead of a force divided they all came at me from the rear and I went down, spilling their feed. Heading back to the house with a coating of mud wasn't unusual and a quick change saw me whisk in hand making a pancake batter as the kids raced down to beat the 8 o'clock rule. If you weren't in the kitchen dressed with shoes and socks by the pips on the radio you went to bed earlier that night. Usually, the rule resulted in silence from upstairs until about 7.55 then a stampede as one or other of the kids realised the time and shouted a shared warning. More often than not all three kids would be in time and the threatened early bed didn't occur.

The kids liked going to their school. It sat elevated next to the shore of Loch Gilp, itself a bite out of Loch Fyne, and looked across the bay to the hills beyond. A modern, recently built structure, it incorporated the pre-5 unit, the Learning Centre, the Primary School and the Secondary School, and was managed by Argyll and Bute Council. Lochgilphead Primary School was a good honest school with a range of children attending. With about 250 pupils across the seven years, it was large enough to see the kids learn the lessons of friendships won and lost but also small enough so no child was lost amongst the masses. Lunch in the school came from the kitchen on the premises and with such a large campus meals started for the primary school

at 11.45 with the aim of having children through quickly so the larger secondary school had time to do the same.

When your child started at the school you were invited to join them for their first school lunch, and it was always nice to meet the dinner ladies who looked after the children every day. I encouraged my children to take a school lunch despite the cost of £2.00 because I saw it as an opportunity for them to choose from a menu and to sit with their friends, neither of which they could do at home. Our family meals were always eaten round the table, sometimes early, sometimes late, depending on which after school activities were going on. As the kids grew and found different things to enjoy it was becoming the only chance we all got to be in the same room at the same time.

Rebecca would tell us what she could about her day. We were all very used to patient confidentiality and even a busy day in the hospital could leave her with little she was able to share. The kids on the other hand were always full of news and it was like chairing a difficult meeting to make sure each of them was given the chance to tell their story, the joke of the day or the latest drama from the school playground.

Dinnertime was also my showcase, my opportunity to share the hard work of my day and of my year. On the plate was my contribution to the family and it was always discussed. The vegetables had either come from the allotment space we had fenced off from the deer or from the 35ft polytunnel that extends our short Scottish growing season. The kids started lots of the vegetables from seed on the windowsills, and it was a common call from the kitchen before dinner for a handful of this or that from the garden. Most of the meat was raised here and we could tell the difference between lamb and hogget and between Berkshire and Tamworth pork.

Sitting down to a casserole of neck of lamb that evening, the sinking of the Titanic was still the hot topic at the table. Work on the project had continued for Martha and she was bubbling over with excitement telling us how she had written a newspaper article like a real journalist on the sinking.

"I want to write like that every day, Dad," she said.

"Every day?" I queried.

"Yes every day because that's what real journalists do for

newspapers. You have to tell everyone what happened. They won't know so you have to tell them the truth. It's easier than writing a story because you don't have to make it up and you get published and you put your name next to it."

I'd rather give the kids time than money and here was a chance to support Martha to do something of her own making.

There was nothing unusual about a big idea coming out around the dinner table. Neither Polly nor Joe batted an eyelid but Rebecca gave me a smile and an encouraging nod. The relationship between Martha and me was probably the most strained in the family. Her world was an emotional one, rich in feelings, friends and drama. Woven into her day at school were threads of friendship struggles that pulled at her own happiness. To be a best friend was important to Martha and she prided herself in that role. Being rejected and replaced could overtake all the good things in her day. Martha and I were blind to the causes of each other's anger. She would, like her mum, shrug at a broken chair, car or computer. I would be visualising the tools, the parts, the awkward laying on my back and the skinned knuckles. To me, repairing a car was a drama that repairing a friendship was not. The only way I could get close to understanding her feelings was to remember the Friday nights when I was her age when, despite my efforts, I was not rewarded with a place on the rugby team. So an opportunity to help Martha write every day was more than an educational project. It was a chance to come together.

"Do you know what a blog is, Martha?" I asked between mouthfuls of casserole. I knew other local primary schools wrote blogs so maybe she'd read them at school.

"No Dad, is it a sort of book?"

"It's not a book but it is something you read. A blog is like a diary. You write it as often as you like, every day even, and you publish it on the internet so anyone can read it. Loads of famous people keep blogs. You can write it on anything you want."

"Does Selena Gomez have a blog?"

"You'll have to look."

Martha leapt to the computer in the corner knowing she had rare permission to use it during a meal.

"She does, she does!"

Martha went quiet as she read the latest news.

I'd never kept a blog but I'd read a lot, from those of a ferryman living off the grid to a crofting pig keeper. I showed them to Martha and asked her what she liked about them. She really enjoyed the blogs we found that had photos.

"What would you write about?" I asked.

"About my school dinners, because I have them every day so I would have something to write about every day and I can show you why I am hungry when I come home."

And so it began. Martha spent the rest of the evening looking at blogs. Together we looked at what she enjoyed about each and a pattern emerged. It was blogs with photos and blogs with ratings that she liked.

"Look Dad, his commute to work on his bike got three stars today and no car doors opened on him. Better than yesterday."

We moved and sat on the sofa with the laptop firmly on Martha's knees.

"Fancy giving it a go, Martha? Not going to be easy to write every day with Brownies and swimming and athletics."

"I'll do it. I'll do it about my dinner. I'll take a photo, rate it and write about it."

So that evening I wrote a letter to her class teacher explaining how Martha wanted to write a blog, that she would like to do it about her school dinners and could she please bring a camera into school. I was sure there wouldn't be a problem. Common sense hadn't left our school and as parents we can take pictures and videos at concerts and plays. Sure enough a couple of days later the head teacher gave me a call.

"Is that Dave?"

"Yes it is, Mrs Stankey," I said, finding it hard to switch to her first name.

"The blog thing is ok. I've checked with the catering department and they say it's fine. Can you make sure you oversee Martha writing it please, and the photos are just to contain her food. She can't have any people in the photos. Other than that, have fun."

"That's great. Thank you. Martha is looking forward to it and I'll let you know the website address."

That evening Martha and I sat down to set up the blog. I managed to wrestle the laptop onto my lap from hers. I had no idea how hard it would be or how much it would cost to set up a blog but with more than 156 million blogs online according to Wikipedia we weren't going to be the first.

"Looks like you need an email address," I said. "And what would you like to call your blog? We need a name. Something to say what the blog's about."

"No More," she suggested.

"No more?"

"Yes, no more because there are never seconds."

I typed 'no more' into the box.

"Sorry love, someone's using that already. It's got to be different to everyone else's."

"Never Seconds then."

I typed in 'never seconds' and it was available. It needed one word for the web address and so NeverSeconds it was. Questions kept popping up as we continued down the set up process and we just tapped in our ideas. Finally it asked us about the author.

"Martha Payne," she typed.

"No no no. It can't be your real name."

"But it's my blog. Journalists have their name in the newspapers."

So launched a discussion about online safety. Joe had recently had a talk in school from a police officer about keeping safe online and he explained it in eleven-year-old boy's speak.

"If you use your real name unkind people can find you and pretend they know you or Mum and Dad and trick you. You don't tell people anything. You don't tell them where you live or where you go to school and you use a pee-sue-denim."

"You mean a pseudonym. The p is silent."

"Yeah one of them," said Joe.

So ten minutes after starting to set up the blog it was done and no money was spent. We'd settled on NeverSeconds. blogspot.co.uk. 'One pupil's daily dose of school dinners' was the description, and Martha was to be known as Veg, or as she put it:

'My dad says I should call myself Veritas Ex Gustu, truth from tasting in Latin but who knows Latin? You can call me Veg.'

MONDAY 30TH APRIL 2012

Eating batteries

Not me, my camera! My best laid plans to take a photo of my school lunch everyday was ruined by a battery eating camera. So no pic of my Shepherd's pie. Tomorrow I hope normal service will resume and I will begin my blog properly, no more false starts!

Every post will have a pic and a list!

Food-o-meter- Out of 10 a rank of how great my lunch was!
Mouthfuls- How else can we judge portion size!
Courses- Starter/main or main/dessert
Health Rating- Out of 10, can healthy foods top the food-o-meter?
Price- Currently £2 I think, its all done on a cashless catering card
Pieces of hair- It wont happen, will it?

Now I really am looking forward to lunch tomorrow,

VEG

Monday 30th April

The first post was up!

Martha was really frustrated with her camera, as she had been keen to show me her lunch. With no photo she'd taken the opportunity to work out the ratings system she wanted to use with each post. We were starting to establish our writing routine. She settled down on the sofa with the laptop and went to NeverSeconds. It was over to me for the password and then click on 'New Post'. Without a pencil to chew Martha looked over the screen, down the garden to the field beyond, a 1000 yard gaze as she composed her thoughts. Sometimes the words would come quickly and whole sentences would be typed rapidly. Other times it would be word-by-word sentence building. But that first day was quick. She knew what she wanted to rate, the possible scores and the names of the categories.

"Pieces of hair?" I asked her.

"Yes Dad. I found a hair. It was really long."

"Like yours you mean."

"It wasn't mine Dad, it was mixed in with my dinner."

"Well maybe that should be the last category for some fun. Are you going to put the rest in order of importance?"

Writing with Martha brought back great memories. With the kids old enough to be independent readers we no longer threw the cushions in the corner, grabbed a book and settled down for some reading. I'd spent hours in that corner, arms aching from holding the book in the one position that all three kids could see it. That wiggle that the kids used to move and mould me into the perfect cuddle position, while sucking their thumbs and getting an elbow in my ribs! Books were everywhere in our house and our favourites were deservedly dog-eared from

enjoyment. The laptop couldn't take the same abuse as the paperbacks but we needed to sit close to see the screen and as she wrote, I helped in the same way I did when she was learning to read. When she struggled on a word we talked. When she queried the red line that appeared I explained it was a spelling error. When she wanted to move the ratings around I explained how to copy and paste.

"Wow that's cool, Dad. Look!" and 'Martha is awesome' was pasted so many times it filled the screen. Once she had mastered the art of highlighting and deleting she was left with her first post.

"Read it one more time before you hit the 'publish' button," I suggested. "Anyone can read it once it's on the blog."

"Even Granny and Grandpa?"

"Yes, and your aunts and uncles and your teacher and they can leave comments on the bottom by clicking that button."

"Do you think they will? Do you think anyone will read it?"

"Sure they will, love. Sure they will."

NeverSeconds One primary school pupil's daily dose of school dinners.

TUESDAY 8TH MAY 2012

I'm back! Many camera failures have stopped me blogging but Dad said I could borrow his camera. I think he's quite shocked at the pictures though.

The first pic is from last week and the second from today. The pizza in the first pic was alright but I'd have enjoyed more than 1 croquet. I'm a growing kid and I need to concentrate all afternoon and I cant do it on 1 croquette. Do any of you think you could?

Food-o-meter- 6/10
Mouthfuls- forgot to count but not enough!
Courses- main/dessert
Health Rating- 4/10
Price- £2
Pieces of hair- 0!

Today's meal was on the menu as Cheeseburger and ice cream/biscuit but as you can see I got an ice lolly. I prefer ice cream. I wish they had stuck to the menu. I did get 2 croquettes though only 3 pieces of cucumber when I said no thanks to the peas.

Food-o-meter- 7/10
Mouthfuls- eating and counting and chatting to friends is hard!
Courses- main/dessert
Health Rating- 2/10
Price- £2
Pieces of hair- 0!

The good thing about this blog is Dad understands why I am hungry when I get home. Today he made a Banana Loaf, shame I don't like bananas, see I am not perfect!

VEG

Tuesday 8th May

With no luck on Martha's camera battery issues the only option was to lend Martha our family digital camera. It was a tough camera, bought because it could be taken underwater and dropped, things that happened regularly to our cameras both in a planned and an unplanned way, so I reckoned it would survive a primary school. With instructions to keep it in her bag other than to take the photo of her dinner she was away to school as usual. In fact she took the photo and kept the camera in her bag all weekend. It wasn't until she had taken a second photo on Tuesday that she reminded me about her blog. I pulled the camera files onto the laptop and open them. Joe and Polly gathered round for a look. I gasped when I saw them and turned to look at the kids. Tellingly, they hadn't batted an eyelid.

"I can see why you are hungry after school then."

"Exactly, Dad. Told you," said Martha.

"Couldn't you have had more than three bits of cucumber?"

"No you can't," interrupted Joe. "You get what you are given. You can't help yourself."

I started uploading the pictures ready to put them on the blog and slid the laptop over to Martha with the blog page open. It struck me that the pictures in front of me were what she had been describing to me for a long time. I had read the menus, I knew that every day she had a choice of salad, a baked potato or one of two hot meals. Only the two hot options changed and I knew that for variety they were her preferred options. I picked up the menu and looked.

"Pizza served with Crunchy Wedges and Seasonal
 Vegetables or Salad"

I ticked the items on her plate off against the menu. All present and correct but the photo showed how much was also missing. It was neither a meal to teach our kids about eating healthily nor about how appetising food can be. I looked at the laptop screen to see what Martha was writing. Frustration was creeping in as her fingers couldn't find the keys fast enough to get her ideas down and each strike of the keyboard was getting louder.

"I'm so slow. I can't do this," she groaned.

"How do you get good at something?" I asked, one of our standard family questions.

"Practice," she answered as she continued to hunt down the letters. Mistakes were appearing underlined in red as the spell-checker did its job.

"Don't worry about spelling now. You can edit at the end. Just get your thoughts down first," I suggested. It must be very daunting for a child to face a jotter, pencil in hand, and know they must fill it with their own words in their own hand, every spelling mistake and correction accompanied by the dark smudge of rubbing out. The blog page on the computer didn't have sheet after sheet to daunt, just one page with colourful margins, images to inspire and no evidence left of any corrections. She finished writing and looked to me for reassurance.

"That's great, Martha! It reads really well. Just some punctuation, then add your ratings and you can publish it."

She added some capitals, corrected spelling mistakes and worked on her ratings.

"I forgot to count my mouthfuls," she worried.

"Then say that. Everyone will understand. You've got to be honest."

She noted down her scores, paused, previewed the post then hit 'publish'. I used my phone to go to Twitter and typed:

'My primary school daughter is blogging her £2 school lunch experiences. I'm speechless. NeverSeconds.blogspot. co.uk Please comment.'

As Martha got on with her homework and I started to prepare tea, my followers on Twitter saw my tweet. Twitter was the

small town experience multiplied, and living in Lochgilphead was great training. Each tweet was that micro conversation I'd had in the aisles of the supermarket, in the swimming pool or the playground by the sea. I have stood in the Post Office queue listening to a customer complain about the hospital and the care she received. She wouldn't have made those comments if she had known the husband of the doctor in question was behind her. Twitter was like having the world stand in that same queue with me, and I knew that if I didn't want to be overheard I shouldn't put it on Twitter.

Beeping from my pocket my phone started to tell me people were replying to my tweet. The beeping became almost constant. The tweet had been repeated, retweeted, and shared again and again. The questions directed to me were pouring in. By 8.20pm, three and a half hours after my first tweet, my Twitter account was trending in the UK and the blog had been visited over 10,000 times. I tried to keep up and replied when I could.

@MikeTonge @newsmary @meeware not fake. My daughter took the pics and wrote it. Tue May 08 18:56:35

@pannusf10 thanks. She had 3 hits at 5pm.9000 now. Tue May 08 20:11:24

@benbarden not at all. Kudos to school for giving her permission to do it. Tue May 08 20:45:34

@isaac_lewis we read together and yes write together it was a thing to do together, then I saw pics and it became about food. Tue May 08 20:47:28

@skinoverbone school gave permission for pics and blog think fair to talk to them before naming. Tue May 08 21:12:38

@virginiamoffatt @BerwickBabs @Jack be great if @jamieoliver encouraged kids all over UK to blog their lunches. Tue May 08 21:19:32

@LunchItPunchIt aye its straight up. Helped along way of course, setting up etc needed an email address! Definitely written together. Tue May 08 22:46:15

Some tweets were uncomfortable, accusing us of making a fake blog. I replied to as many as I could between scouts drop off and pick up, the bedtime routine and stories. I wanted to reply to everyone, it was only polite, but the messages came in so quickly I couldn't read them all let alone reply. Already people wanted the school named. The information miners were on the case and from my Twitter profile they had pinned us down to Argyll. The tweeters were helping me understand the range of reactions the blog was going to generate. Twitter was my window to the future and that night, replying to tweets, I learnt some principles that were to stand us in great stead in the coming months. I was later to bed than usual and under the door of the girls room came the telltale ribbon of light. Opening the door silently I found Martha asleep, bedside light on and book in hand. Slipping her bookmark in for her I kissed her forehead, wondering whether more people would have read her blog by morning than had read the book by her side.

WEDNESDAY 9TH MAY 2012

When I got up this morning Dad told me my blog had 25000 hits so I thought I'd better not forget to count my mouthfuls!

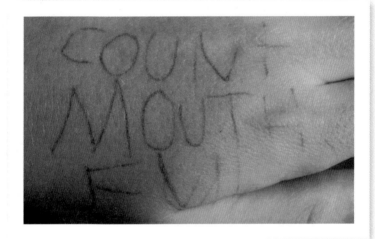

There was an 's' on my thumb but it rubbed off! My photo is a wee bit dark, I've mastered the computer but not my camera!

Today's dinner was carrot and coriander soup followed by mince pasta. I did remember my mouthfuls but as the soup was so hot I burnt my mouth and had to take many little sips! The soup was brilliant. We don't have Carrot and coriander soup very often but its the first time I've tried it and I love it! The mince pasta was the same as spaghetti bolognese but with different shaped pasta and more sweetcorn than last time. I dont know why they call it mince pasta and not just spagbol!

Food-o-meter- 8/10
Mouthfuls- 64 small hot ones
Courses- starter/main
Health Rating- 5/10
Price- £2
Pieces of hair- still in the clear

My blog has had 42000 hits now and I hope one of them was Jamie Oliver!

VEG

Wednesday 9th May

Lambing was taking its toll. I'd been up twice checking for our last ewe to lamb. She was old, experienced and reliable, but still needed an eye kept on her and so twice in the night I had gone to the fields. Putting the big lamp back on charge gave me the chance to check the computer. Hits and comments were accumulating rapidly. I got back to bed from my dawn check and Rebecca muttered, "Everything ok?"

"The ewe's showing no signs. The blog's taken off though."

I felt her stiffen next to me.

"How many?"

"20,000 and climbing."

She was silent for a second.

"You should tell the school first thing. Send a letter."

She drifted back to sleep. Maybe it was her years as an on-call doctor that let her go from sleep to alert to sleep so easily. No such luck for me and I lay awake pondering the 20,000.

I was chuffed for Martha. She'd had an idea, shared it and published her first post but of the thousands who had read it would be those few, the teachers and dinner ladies, whose reactions would be important to Martha. No one could be happy to be part of the system serving a nine year old those dinners surely and the dinner ladies at the end of the chain couldn't be the ones to blame. They prepared the food they were told to prepare and served the quantities they were told to serve yet clearly something had gone astray and Martha had shown that to a lot of people. Embarrassment was a strange emotion and there were some moments in my life that I couldn't help but physically wince at when I remembered them. Martha had embarrassed a lot of people by blogging her dinner and I wondered how they

would react. Soon enough it was breakfast and time for another letter to her teacher.

'Dear Mr Maddox,
Martha's blog has had over 25,000 hits overnight. I thought I ought to let you know.'

"Happy with that Martha?" I asked, showing her the letter.

"Will I get into trouble, Dad?" She looked really nervous putting the letter in her bag.

"You've done nothing wrong. You asked for permission. I think your teacher will be really impressed."

She gave me a hard look.

"I want to take my photo and blog today. I like it."

I took the camera and placed it in her bag. I was pleased that we had something to do together. I was looking forward to it. We didn't give the kids a lot of stuff. We spent time not money on them and it was easy with Joe and Polly. As the eldest and keen on his biking I only had to suggest to Joe a cycle or swim and he was up for it. We'd lose an hour in the woods exploring the mountain bike trails regularly. With Polly I needed to suspend reality. Her favourite toy was an old saddle that she scrubbed and cleaned for hours before polishing and throwing it over the back of the sofa so she could ride every day. For Martha there hadn't been that one thing we shared together and the blog was starting to give us that time. I gave her a cuddle as she dashed out the door. Unusually she didn't squirm.

After a couple of hours with the stock on the smallholding it was definitely time for a coffee. The computer was in the corner of the room next to the kitchen and I sat down to look at the comments submitted. Anyone could write a response to the blog but they didn't go straight onto the web. Instead the comments were stored and I moderated them before publishing. Folk were being really kind in writing their encouragement to her and showing their support.

Lorraine9

Well done "Veg" (great pseudonym)! What a fantastic blog, well written and with brilliant photographs. I'm appalled though that your school thinks they can get away with giving growing children such rubbish food. I hope your blog will make a difference and shame them and other schools across the country to do much better! I'm going to tweet about this right now. All power to you!

Already the blog was being treated as a campaign for better school meals. Martha certainly could campaign. Her most recent had been for a later bedtime but she hadn't had such intentions with the blog, had she? The phone rang. Looking at the clock I expected it to be the school but it wasn't.

"Hi, is this Martha's Dad?"

"Who's calling please?"

"I'm calling from the Daily Record."

A phone call from Scotland's largest selling newspaper.

"Can I call you back? Bit busy lambing just now. Thanks."

Never had I been so grateful to have the excuse of lambing. How did they get my number? How did they know my name? I'll never know but it was clear it was going to be the first of many calls. The phone rang again.

"Hi Dave, it's the swimming pool," said the voice. "We're getting lots of calls asking for your contact details from newspapers and TV."

"Oh right. Could you not hand them out please."

"We haven't done, just wanted to check. They are finding you on YouTube at the march."

Back in 2009 I had organised a march in Lochgilphead to support the community swimming pool, which was under threat of closure. The phone rang again, this time a friend I swam with.

"Hi Dave, how's it going?" she said.

"Bit odd really. Getting some calls about Martha's blog."

"That's why I am calling. You know I write for the papers sometimes. Do you want me to pass your number onto a friend? People try their whole lives to trend on Twitter and Martha's blog is. You'd better speak to someone or they'll be at your door."

"You'd recommend it?"

"Don't give it away, Dave. You should make something for Martha out of this."

It hadn't occurred to me that a paper would be willing to pay. I was more concerned about keeping Martha protected than money.

"OK. Who'd you recommend?"

"Daily Mail will look after you. Do it once in the right place and the pressure will be off."

"OK. Pass it along. Thanks. Getting a bit nervous now."

"Don't worry it'll be fine. Speak soon."

My hands were shaking. I turned back to the computer and looked again at the photos and Martha's writing. The photos stared back. It really was no wonder that the press wanted more. The phone rang again. It was Paul Harris from the Daily Mail. He asked after Martha, how she was, did she know that a storm had erupted? We chatted about her asking to write and choosing a blog about her school dinners.

It was still a few hours until Martha was due to be collected from school and the Mail were keen to send a photographer but I had to speak to Rebecca and Martha before we could agree. That wasn't a problem and the chat turned to exclusivity and figures. We weren't ones to seek the fast buck and it seemed there was a standard fee for this kind of story and I agreed without negotiation.

That afternoon was a constant stream of calls. Our number was out there but having made an arrangement with Paul it was much easier for me to say that we had a deal with the Mail and the journalists were respectful of that. Twitter was now being used by journalists to make contact as well. Years of meeting new people daily in my instructor days were helping. I didn't mind chatting to new people on the phone or on Twitter and the approach stood us in good stead. Taking time to help them get their facts straight was well spent and the articles that came from those I had spent time with were more accurate than those I couldn't. I was finding the people I spoke with not to be the ogres that I might have expected. They were grateful for my time and every conversation I hoped conveyed the message we were a normal family and not one out for fame or fortune.

There was nothing unusual about picking the kids up from school. No teacher waiting for a quiet word, no letter coming home in Martha's bag. I had been expecting both. It was to be the usual hurried evening of homework and then Brownies, but tonight the extra time to write the blog and meet the photographer was added in. Martha's determination could swing towards a fun evening getting loads done or to fighting me every step of the way. Added to the mix, it was her mum's night to be out so the safety cushion she usually threw between Martha and me was not to be available either. I'd honed my parenting skills on Joe, a happy go lucky kind of boy who'd just rolled with the plans. When I was nine, I was in a boys' boarding school where doing as you were told meant doing it immediately or facing a strict punishment. Martha was no boy and home was no boarding school so my experiences to date hadn't been the best preparation.

"Hey Martha, how do you fancy getting your photo taken by a proper photographer?"

I explained that the number of hits on the blog was now 42,000 and a newspaper was writing a story about it. I showed her an article that had already appeared in an online newspaper, The Huffington Post, and she read it thoroughly.

"I'll speak to them and do the photos if you want," she said.

"It's up to you really but I think it's a good idea. Paul is very nice. You can't say anything wrong."

Martha tipped her head to one side. I looked back at her wondering how a nine year old would process it all.

"Will I be famous tomorrow?"

"Do you want to be?"

"No, I want to see my friends. Famous people don't have proper friends."

"Oh I think they do. Famous people just keep their friends secret."

"Can I still go to Brownies?"

With the news it would all be done before Brownies she was happy and took to the trampoline to celebrate. The photographer duly arrived and snapped away. Martha here, Martha there, Martha with laptop, no laptop, Martha and Dad and one special photo.

"Just for the family," he said as he took a portrait shot of Martha on the sofa. That picture was the one that appeared around the world.

NeverSeconds One primary school pupil's daily dose of school dinners.

THURSDAY 10TH MAY 2012

Big news, I have gone viral! 105,000 people have visited my blog and thanks to all of you. Even bigger news my dad got a tweet from Jamie Oliver!

"Shocking but inspirational blog. Keep going, Big love from Jamie x"

I am really glad he looked in and it has put a smile on my face. I was a bit nervous going to school but everyone was great and I'm glad I haven't upset anybody.

I love Mexican food and today's Chicken Fajita was very nice and enjoyable. It was stuffed with salsa and chicken and served with garlic bread. I got sent back for salad as I missed it first time round!

Food-o-meter- 8/10
Mouthfuls- forgot to write on hand, forgot to count.
Courses- main/dessert
Health Rating- 6/10
Price- £2
Pieces of hair- none, not even one of mine.

Looking forward to tomorrow's menu,

VEG

Thursday 10th May

By the time I got back from the newsagent Rebecca was up and we opened the newspaper together.

"You didn't even change from your work trousers," was Rebecca's first comment, "but the article is alright isn't it?"

I read the article carefully looking for inaccuracies.

"It seems fine. Wonder how the school and council will react."

The decision to talk to the press was a response to the growing coverage. People wanted to see the little girl who wrote about her dinner and by cooperating with a paper we'd satisfied the public demand, or so we thought. Everyone had expectations and Rebecca, maybe used to managing patients' expectations, had the language to manage ours as well.

"What do you want to get out of this?" she asked as we sat, coffees in hand, before the kids got up.

"Be nice to see the kids getting a decent school dinner. She's really enjoying writing it and I enjoy the time with her. She gave me a huge hug after she published it last night. Not sure she liked doing the photos."

"But where do you think it's going?"

I had been thinking about this from about 2am to 5am. I'd not managed sleep between ewe checks just because my head was whirling.

"The council will get involved. They'll come in and focus on the good. It'll be all about 'how great and supportive Argyll schools are to encourage and allow a nine-year-old's project. Isn't it wonderful it's being recognised around the world. Yes, there's clearly an issue but thanks to Veg we can work it out together'. The council will phone today."

It was still before 7am as I poured my second coffee and the phone went. There was a picture of Martha in another paper. I looked online and there was a family photograph of a seven-year-old Martha staring back at me. I recognised it immediately. It was on a Thames river bus outside the Tower of London. We were alongside Traitor's gate. How appropriate. That picture scared us. Someone must have sold it to the papers. Rebecca started checking her Facebook account to see if the photo was there. It was not on either of our accounts. That instinct to protect our wee ones was so powerful. I could see Rebecca prickling with rage.

"How could they? How could someone give them that picture?" She crumpled into her chair.

"It won't happen again. There are pictures out there now. That's why we did the photos but we couldn't have done them any quicker."

It was to be one of the low points of the whole story for us. Not just because of the photo but because of the way I handled it. Leaping in to defend Martha, I assumed a family member had sold it. I was wrong and discovered too late it had been lifted from a photo service I used to Tweet from my phone. I had taken the picture and a setting on my share options had sent it to Twitpic and there it had been for two years waiting to be tracked down by a paper. As we pondered the unwanted photo we didn't realise that the Daily Mail story was being discussed on breakfast television. Facebook friends started posting they'd seen us on TV. As we got ready for the school run we were blissfully unaware that the story was being run in every national newspaper and was to appear across all the television networks during the day.

My mobile phone was starting to sound like a crazed drum machine as it emitted beeps for incoming tweets, emails, text messages and missed calls. It sat ignored in my pocket, as our last ewe was doing her thing and I was dealing with a cracking pair of young lambs. Handling anything after spraying the lambs' navels with iodine is impossible until you've scrubbed your hands. Getting back to normality was really important, even just for half an hour. Martha's NeverSeconds was starting to consume my time endlessly. Kindly, Paul at the Daily Mail

checked with us before sharing our details with ITV Daybreak. I'd just had a message from Rebecca that calls and emails were now coming into the hospital trying to track us down. Things certainly didn't seem to be calming down. By going into the behind the scenes statistics area on the blog I was able to see which links were bringing visitors to the blog. Newspapers around the world were reporting the story online and in print. A map of the world highlighted which countries were hitting the blog in numbers. Spain, Italy, America, Japan and Taiwan were top of the list. If it was big news in the UK it was bigger news worldwide.

The press discussing the blog was one thing. Twitter was another. I never read the comments on the newspaper online articles. The Daily Mail article was heading for almost 600 comments but I felt much more at home on Twitter. The blog was Martha's place to write, Twitter was mine. As a way of gauging public reaction it's second to none. Whilst 140 characters is a challenge it has been mastered by many and the thoughts shared on NeverSeconds helped me keep on top of the issues. It was my place to encourage and share ideas.

I knew Martha was benefitting from her experience of blogging. She was learning so many knew skills. Her typing was already noticeably quicker and I had no doubt she could move the photo files from SD card to website by herself if needed. She was taking pride in her work, pausing to preview and edit her sentences before publishing, changing whole phrases that didn't mean what she wanted to say. More importantly, she was considering carefully what she wrote and sticking to the truth before sharing the experience as she saw it through her own eyes. When Jamie Oliver sent her a message of support it became news in itself.

Jamie Oliver ✔
@jamieoliver

@ballibeg neverseconds.blogspot.co.uk
Shocking but inspirational blog. Keep going,
Big love from Jamie x

← Reply ⇄ Retweet ★ Favorite

Journalists now wanted to speak to her because Jamie Oliver
had tweeted to her. ITV Daybreak wanted us to meet Jamie
on their sofa on Monday morning. America wanted live TV
link ups. The BBC wanted us to do an interview for You and
Yours and in amongst all the attention it was passed on to me
by a journalist that Argyll and Bute Council had replied to his
questions with this:

> 'Young people make a choice from at least two meals and
> salad, vegetable, yoghurt and cheese options are available
> each day. An unlimited amount of bread and salad are
> available to all pupils who wish to take them and fruit is
> also always available.'

It certainly would be news to my kids that they could have
more. No signs were up to tell the kids this and they received
no encouragement. Surely it would be better to confirm this
with the children in the school rather than with the press? I was
glad things were going to improve for the children at school and
that the council was finding time to talk to the press. It was just
such a shame they couldn't find time to talk to us.

The journalist was very surprised that no positive spin was
being put out. No celebration of one of their pupil's success-
ful blog. No 'we'll look into this and if there is a problem we'll
rectify it'. The council's approach was to influence ours. We
accepted the interview request from the BBC You and Yours
programme and after a polite chat with a reporter at the school
gates we visited the small BBC cupboard studio in Oban. We
sat waiting with headphones on, having pressed the buttons

43

that the note on the wall told us to, and miraculously in our heads was the voice of Julian Worricker. Martha told her story for herself to be broadcast on Monday.

Friday 11th May

The problem with teaching your kids that life is about experiences and not about money is that when you get offered an experience money can't buy you want to take it, or at least I did.

ITV Daybreak had invited us to the sofa in London on Monday to meet Jamie Oliver and feelings in the house were mixed. I thought as trips went it was pretty special. Daybreak had listened to us when we explained we did not want to single Martha out from the family as receiving special attention and consequently they had invited us all to travel down on Sunday, stay in a hotel near the studios and then join them on the set. Martha was ahead of me.

"Will I have to say anything? Will they ask me questions? I don't like questions."

Martha had shown in her posts that she was thoughtful but time was her friend on the laptop. She developed her ideas from writing them down and reading them. The experience of the BBC booth in Oban had unsettled her. She'd got no clues from the face or body language of Julian, just his voice in her head and there had been awkward silences when she had started to speak again just as he did.

"I want to be a journalist because they ask questions and don't answer them," she said firmly.

With exquisite timing, Good Morning Scotland on the radio cut to the voice of Kaye Adams announcing the details of her morning radio phone in show. It was to include NeverSeconds. Martha looked at her feet, twisting her heels. I couldn't guess her feelings from her movement but her Mum and I knew we'd never seen her behave like this before. Rebecca wrapped her in a cuddle and Polly dived in too.

"People are talking about school dinners again because of your blog," Rebecca said to Martha as they rocked gently.

"It's a good thing, Martha," I added, joining the cuddle. "You've drawn attention to something important by writing about it. Well done."

"I want to meet Jamie Oliver but I'm worried I'll say something silly or I won't be able to answer a question. They won't understand my accent. My friends will watch it and if it's bad they'll laugh at me."

"I don't think we should go. It's too far to travel, too early to get up and Dad will be grumpy because he'll be shattered," said Rebecca.

"I'm never grumpy," I complained, much to the mirth of the girls. Joe, who had evaded my attempt to drag him into the cuddle, was bouncing. "You're so grumpy!"

It was great to hear the whole family laughing. I left the cuddle to answer the phone. It was the Call Kaye programme on BBC Radio Scotland inviting me on.

"It's very kind," I thanked them, "but no thanks." I was starting to feel talked out and resorted to economy of words.

Every time I spoke to a journalist I was giving an interview. I could tell from their voices that the phone was wedged between head and shoulder, or it had that distant sound that comes from headset microphones. I could hear the keys on the computer tapping away and naturally I'd fall into their rhythm, waiting patiently for the drumming to stop before continuing my sentence. But each time I spoke I was putting myself at risk. The next call could be the one when I'd make a slip, let my tiredness get the better of me or fire a broadside attack. Live radio was a step too far. I'd gone from taking every opportunity to support Martha to accepting that she didn't need it.

Across the world children were responding to her blog. Emails of school dinners were arriving with photos and ratings. Teachers and politicians were tweeting the blog's praises. A child was being listened to and more children wanted to be listened to with her. They were all her supporters and it was as if the internet had picked her up and wrapped its multitude of protective arms around her.

I got on with my day as usual but deliberately avoided

Food-o-meter- 8/10
Mouthfuls- I must take a pad to keep tally!
Courses- starter/main
Health Rating- 6/10
Price- £2
Pieces of hair- 1 (under the cucumber)

I'd really like it if other people could send in their photos of their school dinners and rate them the way I do. I'll put them on my blog. Please send them to NeverSeconds@gmail.com

VEG

Monday 14th May

The radio interview that Martha and I had recorded for BBC Radio 4's You and Yours was aired at lunchtime and I recorded it for Martha. I hadn't told her about the interview that Malcolm MacFadyen had given and she was excited about hearing us talk.

"Did you recognise my voice?" she asked.

"Of course, I sound really funny though," I replied as we pulled up to the house.

"You always sound funny. You don't sound Scottish at all."

She wasn't wrong. Growing up in Lincolnshire doesn't give you much of a Scottish accent. We gathered round the stereo and I started the recording. Martha played at covering her ears as she heard herself speak about why she had started her blog and what she liked and didn't like about her food. We'd both answered the questions put to us honestly and clearly and I was really pleased that Martha had managed so well. We were followed by Jayne Murphy, introduced as being responsible for school meals in Argyll and Bute. She expressed surprise as she felt the pictures showed only half a meal; that lettuce, cherry tomatoes and watercress and many other items were also available. Martha's photographs were, in Jayne's opinion, a reflection of Martha's choices. She was clearly taking the same line as Malcolm MacFadyen. I watched Martha as the interview went on. There was nothing I could do to protect her from the words she was hearing. I could see the tears welling up in her eyes as she dipped her head into her hands.

"That's so unfair. That's not right. I have everything I'm allowed. You're only allowed veg or salad not both and you get what you're given."

"Are you absolutely sure?" I asked.

Joe and Polly backed her up.

"I've never seen watercress ever at school," Joe added.

"She probably doesn't agree with you Martha that some of the food isn't nice either," I suggested.

"That's just Martha's opinion," said Joe, "but it's a fact we can't get more. It says on the menu veg or salad you can't get both. Look."

Joe showed me the menu and it did say just that.

"I don't think the lady would lie. I think there's confusion somewhere," I offered to the kids. "Maybe you are allowed it but you don't ask."

"We're not, Dad. We're just not," Martha said and she stormed off to the lounge and picked up the laptop. I took Joe to the side.

"This is serious, Joe. It's not a game. You need to be honest with us about what's on offer."

"We are, Dad. We are," he promised.

I sat with Martha and opened up the blog page for her.

"How was your lunch today?" I asked as she started typing.

"There was a hair and there weren't any mini tomatoes or watercress and that's what I am going to tell everyone. I'm going to tell the truth."

Martha had started to develop a structure to her posts. She started with a paragraph of news, and then the photo went in followed by her ratings underneath. I showed her how to look up the number of visitors to the blog in case she wanted to include it.

"Can I say I was on the radio? I want people to hear what that lady said about me."

"Why not. It's probably better to let people listen and make up their own minds. You said things about the food as well remember."

"I will put it in then."

She started to write, dragging the laptop back up when it slid too far down her legs for her to reach the keyboard. I passed her a cushion to even things up. I knew the next day councillors along with staff from the council headquarters had been invited to try the food for themselves. The local press were going along and had asked to meet Martha and me at home afterwards. It was a shame neither my wife nor I was invited to join them all

for lunch at school and I couldn't help but wonder if they were avoiding us after their comments on national radio. It would have been an ideal opportunity to clear up any misunderstandings and move on. I resolved that if the council did not approach us for a chat then we would have to contact them and arrange it.

"What do you think, Dad?"

I read through her post and smiled at her comments on the tomatoes and watercress.

"There's the publish button," I said handing back the mouse.

She slid the pointer over and with a single click sent it online.

TUESDAY 15TH MAY 2012

Today was very different at lunchtime. Dad had already told me beforehand that some people from the Council were coming to lunch with a reporter from our local paper. There was also a new system for ordering food which I'll explain when I understand it more. I didn't see the visitors having lunch but I saw them hovering about and watching us getting served.

For the first time ever I have seen at lunch cherry tomatoes, radishes, carrot and cucumber shreddings. I didn't see any watercress but I may have missed it. I chose macaroni cheese, mashed potato, cucumber and peppers. The macaroni cheese is always good but I could always eat more. I was asked today for the first time, 'Is that enough for you?'. For my dessert I had red jelly which tasted of strawberries. I liked most of the changes and I hope it will be the same tomorrow.

Food-o-meter- 9/10
Mouthfuls- 33, I took a pad and my pen ran out but I
remembered!
Courses- main/dessert
Health Rating- 6/10
Price- £2
Pieces of hair- 0

Thank you for all your pictures. Today's is from Pol Elia
from Spain. I like the way the the veg is mixed in with the
stew. Ours always come seperately.

Pol Elia's ratings are,

Food-o-meter- 7/10
Health Rating- 5/10
Price- €2.06, which is £1.64
Pices of hair- 1

Tomorrow I will remember to look for the watercress!

VEG

Tuesday 15th May

It was great to be getting a full night's sleep again with lambing over. It had been a good year for our small flock and our seven breeding ewes had had thirteen lambs between them. The lambs were doing well under the watchful eye of Pedro, our guard llama, and we hadn't lost any so far to illness or fox. Mornings were more leisurely and I had time for a longer walk with the dog or even a run before waking the kids.

My new routine was to leave my phone downstairs on charge instead of leaving it in my pocket by the bed. With the global interest in the blog we were receiving dozens of emails overnight. Most concerning press had MEDIA REQUEST in the subject line and one caught my eye as I made coffee. From a Japanese TV station we had an invitation to travel to Tokyo and join a class in school there to blog a Japanese school lunch. They had certainly done their research as the itinerary included our travel time to Glasgow for our connecting flight to Heathrow. For a moment I could imagine us all in the hustle and bustle of Tokyo, exploring the school together and Martha making friends over lunch. I was finding it harder to remain grounded than Martha, and Rebecca's calm reality check was needed. I replied with a 'thank you for your kind offer but...'

The lack of official communication from the school was becoming more and more awkward until it was explained quietly that the staff had been instructed not to speak to us. It was great to know we had support on the quiet even if officially it could not be offered. Martha had gone off to school recovered from her upset over the radio interview and we had chatted with her before she left about the guests expected at school for dinner that day. With no invitation ourselves we were concerned that

Martha might be under pressure and we had to insist no photographs were to go to print that had been taken of her with various adults. Despite the ban on communications I received a number of text messages from inside the school describing the spread on offer that day as 'incredible' and 'we've never seen anything like it before'. It was very disappointing that the wool was being deliberately pulled over the visitors' eyes.

Speaking at home later that afternoon with one of the journalists who'd also had previous experience of the dinners, the same sentiment was expressed. With behaviour like this it was no wonder the council were insistent that no teacher could talk to the press. Martha shrugged it off but was happy to comment on the new choices and the illusive watercress. She was more excited about the food photos and ratings that were being sent in by children from around the world.

Children were copying her and she loved it. She included the first submitted photo from Spain and commented on the stew. The submissions brought a whole new element to the blog. No longer were Martha's photos standing in splendid isolation but a comparison could be made to another child's, another school's and another country's school dinner. The differences were apparent immediately in both quality and price. We were learning together now. Ingredients that were unfamiliar had to be googled and if that failed we waited until comments on the blog revealed all. We started tracking the kids on a globe and soon I would be timing her to find that day's location and she would include the number of seconds on the blog. It was thrilling that other children were picking up cameras and using them as a tool to focus their minds on the food in front of them. NeverSeconds was becoming a place for children to share and broaden their knowledge of food and it was wonderful to watch Martha's horizons stretch from Lochgilphead out across Scotland and beyond.

WEDNESDAY 16TH MAY 2012

The new things from yesterday, the radishes, the mini tomatoes and the shreddings weren't to be seen today. Maybe it was just because my class was last in the queue and I was the last in the school to be served. I was looking forward to the radishes because I have not had one for a while.

If soup is on and some sort of cake and you are having some sort of roll, wrap or sandwich you are allowed to have soup and a cake. The soup today was potato and leek. I really like all the school's soups. My roll was white bread with butter and grated cheese. I am not sure what cheese it is. I had cucumber and lettuce with it. Normally all the cakes are iced but today we had a choice of iced or not. I chose iced!

Food-o-meter- 9/10
Mouthfuls- 29
Courses- starter/main/dessert
Health Rating- 7/10
Price- £2
Pieces of hair- 0

I need more time to understand the band system for ordering, more on that tomorrow. Please can you send in your pics and ratings for your school lunches to NeverSeconds@gmail.com . I'm really keen to compare yours with mine.

VEG

Thursday 17th May

Rebecca was getting concerned about the local reaction to the blog. Working amongst receptionists and nurses at the hospital coupled with being a popular doctor meant she was chatting to far more people a day than I was. There were a range of opinions from those who felt it was a pushy parent driven attempt for fame to those who agreed whole heartedly with what we were doing. I was at the school every day collecting at 3.30pm and chatted happily with the usual crowd of parents as we awaited the charge of the kids out of school. At every opportunity with the press I was highlighting the positives about the quality of the school and its teachers. Martha could not have been happier and all of the kids enjoyed school and looked forward to it.

If my phone was busy I suspected the school's phone was busier. Knowing how hard running a school was, the added work from journalists must have been as much of a strain on them as it was on us. Kindly letters arriving at the school addressed to 'Veg, Food Critic' were handed on to Martha at the end of each day. It was hard explaining to Martha not to open them. We didn't know the senders and I wanted to be the first to see the contents. In fact we never received anything untoward.

The blog's continuing appearance in the papers and on TV around the world gave the appearance we were pushing hard to keep the issue in the headlines. Instead I was turning away requests daily for TV crews to visit our home. Sky, BBC, STV and Channel 5 news had all been in touch along with networks from the USA, Canada, New Zealand, Australia, France, Germany, Spain, Italy and Taiwan. Documentary makers wanted to film footage of Martha's reactions to the press to use in longer programmes to be made at a later date. The BBC One Show had

been in touch to make a section for their show and as with all the requests we politely said no. Our reputation in media circles was as a family that said no and it was considered to be unusual. Whilst I was happy to read Twitter's take on the blog, Rebecca was reading the comments on local websites and newspaper websites, something I refused to do. The reaction she was witnessing was different to the one I was but between us we had a good idea of the depth of feeling it was stirring on all sides of the debate.

"I'm off to meet the council today kids," I said, helping to sort gym kit after breakfast.

"You going to complain about the food?" asked Joe.

"Keener to complain about their comments on the radio I think. We'll have to talk about the food as well but hopefully we'll sort out a plan for the future."

I'd decided a continuing silence between the council and ourselves was in no one's interest. Arrangements were swiftly made and I was fortunate that I was able to ask a local councillor to join us for the meeting, which took place at the council headquarters in Lochgilphead.

Kilmory is an old semi-stately home, added to over the years to accommodate the large number of staff and offices a council needs. Argyll and Bute Council is one of the largest employers in the area and passing along its corridors and staircases I recognised many faces from the town.

I took copies of the menus into the meeting, along with my laptop with the recorded radio interviews on.

I'm not a regular meeting attendee but I was struck by the lack of any person taking notes. Surely a record of our discussion would be useful in the future. I pointed out to both Malcolm MacFadyen and Jayne Murphy that I felt their comments on the radio were erroneous and unfair to Martha. I offered to play the recordings back and go through them in detail but Mr MacFadyen at this point had his head in his hands and I had no wish to further his embarrassment. Figures and documents from the head teacher of the primary school were produced to show she was happy with the dinner service and when I pointed out the incredible spread laid on for the press and visitors Mrs Murphy assured me she had been told that was not the case.

So there we were, four adults sat around a table discussing photographs of Martha's school meals but unable to agree on the facts. They were insistent that the children were able to have more whilst my children, and my contacts in the school, said differently. I asked if there were any signs that maybe the kids had missed. It seemed not. One of the reasons put to me why children weren't having more was that the serving apparatus was taller than the children so they couldn't see it. Common sense should have provided the answers to all these problems, but no solution had been introduced yet. I described the media pressure we were being subjected to and my suggestion of a joint press release, explaining we had discussed the issues and were positively moving forward, was well received. Mr MacFadyen was going to leave the meeting and arrange it for release as soon as possible, which could even be the same day.

We all left the meeting smiling and shaking hands, and I promised to email the 'Voice of Russia' podcast where the meals were being heralded as an attempt to curb the gluttony of the west as an example of the weirder side of the tale. I was very happy with the way it had gone. I had explained our position clearly and demonstrated that we were not keen to keep this in the press. I had received assurances that their comments had not meant to cause offence, that they were sorry that they had and that we could move on cooperatively.

I waited in the rest of the day for the press release to arrive for my approval. It didn't come. Nor did it come the next day or the day after. In fact it never came. It was as if the meeting had never taken place. In itself this was newsworthy. Argyll and Bute were throwing away a golden opportunity to diffuse any press interest with a statement of cooperation between us. Not for the last time the council was snatching defeat from the jaws of success.

Martha came home very excited. I had let slip there was a parcel waiting for her.

"A parcel? Is it big? Is it heavy?"

Kids love receiving anything in the post with their name on and this certainly wasn't going to be a boring birthday card from the bank. Martha bobbed as I fumbled the key into the door.

"Carefully," I suggested as she ripped the package open.

Inside was a book from Jamie Oliver. I knew it was coming but I had left it as a surprise to her.

"It's from Jamie!"

Opening it to the first page there was an inscription to her:

'Dear Martha, great work!! Clever girl, lots of love Jamie, xxx, Keep it up!!'

Martha had already heard Jamie discuss her on ITV Daybreak and he had suggested she should take over from him on school meals. She felt close enough to him from that, in her nine-year-old way, to feel she knew him. The book meant a lot to Martha. So much so that we had to buy her another copy to cook from as she didn't want to damage the one she had been sent. It was funny watching her puff up with pride to have a message from someone who was an inspiration to her, and her resolve to continue her blog hardened because of it.

NeverSeconds One primary school pupil's daily dose of school dinners.

THURSDAY 17TH MAY 2012

My Dad met the council today and its official that we are allowed unlimited salads, fruit and bread! I'm really happy that all of my friends can help themselves to good stuff. This is the message that Jamie Oliver wrote in his Jamie's Great Britain book which he kindly sent to me,

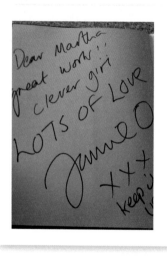

Thanks Jamie, I do intend to keep it up!

Today my lunch was baked potato and cheese. I was given an overload of salad and with the potato it really filled me up and it was hard to finish. The brownie is definitely better than Dads as it has sticky chocolate icing on it. It is crumbs in the photo by the cake, not flies.

Food-o-meter- 6/10
Mouthfuls- 48 (didn't quite finish the salad)
Courses- main/dessert
Health Rating- 9/10
Price- £2
Pieces of hair- 0

Today my blog has become massive in Taiwan and here is a picture sent in by Annie from Taiwan.

She says it is a normal lunch. I don't recognise all the foods but it looks very colourful and tasty!

Tomorrow I'm looking forward to dipping lots of bread in my soup if its on the menu.

VEG

Friday 18th May

"Is it a journalist?" Martha demanded as I passed her the phone.

"Of course not, it's Grandpa John."

Martha took the phone and started wandering around as she spoke with him. We'd been very careful to shield Martha from talking to the press and so despite the constant ringing of the phone it was rarely for her. She was telling Grandpa all about her day at school and what she had done at Dolphins swimming club the evening before.

"We're going to Gigha on Saturday and I'm going to race on my bike," I heard her tell Grandpa. "I'm going to try and beat Mum!"

A trip down the Kintyre peninsula to take the short ferry hop to the island of Gigha was planned for the annual Challenge Gigha day of bike races and running races. Rebecca had better watch her back.

"And I am going to put Mary's Meals on my blog as well," Martha announced to Grandpa. She stopped pacing and listened intently.

I had no idea what John was saying to her but she was smiling and nodding. John first came into contact with Mary's Meals back in 2007 when he heard Tom Farmer, a Scottish entrepreneur, talk about them at a charity event. John and his wife Jane, Martha's maternal grandparents, were inspired to get involved and they had both been volunteers with the charity ever since.

Mary's Meals provided daily meals to chronically hungry children in places of learning. Kids were attracted to the classrooms where they could gain a better future for themselves and their community. The charity also ran a scheme to send backpacks out to children with materials to support them at

school. Grandpa John received collections of backpacks from schools and Joe, Martha and Polly had grown up associating a visit to their grandparents with the chance to help sort these backpacks. Maybe it was the excitement of opening each bag to discover its contents that kept them enthralled but they spent hours helping to organise the bags so each had roughly the same contents so no child would be disappointed when receiving theirs. These backpacks would later be collected and delivered to the Mary's Meals warehouse in Glasgow, ready to be packed up into a shipping container to be sent to a Mary's Meals school somewhere in the world. Joe, Martha and Polly had each sent a couple of backpacks already as part of the scheme and had filled them with notebooks, pencils, towels, toothpaste, toothbrush and a t-shirt.

Martha put the phone back very excited.

"Grandpa thinks it's a great idea because Mary's Meals is about school food for children and so is my blog. I can tell everyone about Charity Children and all the money we raised."

NeverSeconds was being read by about 50,000 people a day and so it would be a great opportunity to tell the world about the Scottish charity from just up the road that was feeding 650,000 children a day at school throughout the world.

Cuddled up in our favourite spot, laptop on knees, Martha began to write her blog. I organised the photograph and whilst the file transferred over she began looking at the Mary's Meals website for more information.

"Dad, look at Mandida. She's from Malawi." Martha was pointing to a photo of a girl on the website. "She's got no parents and sometimes had to go without food for three days but now she gets a Mary's Meal at school. Because she gets a dinner she doesn't have to beg or work so she can go to school. She wants to be a lawyer then president."

"All because of a school dinner. It's great to share it on your blog. Do you know what they eat at school?"

"Mandida eats porridge. Imagine porridge every day for lunch."

"You know I spend £2 a day for your school dinner and the council say it actually costs £3.06 to produce. Mandida's lunch cost 4p and the global average for a Mary's Meal is 6p." I showed

Martha how to find the calculator on the laptop. "The cost of your dinner would have given a school dinner to Mandida and 75 of her friends today."

Martha showed me the photograph of her dinner.

"Where's the watercress?" I joked with her.

"I got extra veg for the first time today, peas, and one was black!" She screwed up her nose.

I looked at Martha's photo. I had no idea how a tiny burger, nine chips, extra peas and a cake could cost £3.06 to produce, nor could I understand why a nation with a problem of heart disease, obesity and diabetes could allow any child to have that for lunch. As long as junk food was available then children would choose it. Whenever an advert break started on television we insisted the sound was turned off. It was automatic now for the children to do this but despite our best efforts they still had junk food sold to them.

With the London Olympics around the corner the sponsoring companies were beginning to ramp up their advertising. Alongside images of the world's best athletes were images of some of the world's unhealthiest foods. I wondered how many gold medal winners would have trained on a diet of burgers, fries and sugar filled drinks. Of course it was easy for the council to blame the children for their choices but what chance did a child have to learn about healthy food when advertisers were selling them the opposite? School was the opportunity to introduce children to a range of tasty healthy foods. A visit to the dining hall was more than a pit stop to refuel, and should have been treated as another lesson. A burger and chips had been given to Martha with the approval of the Scottish Government because it met their guidelines, and I winced as she rated it 9/10 on the food-o-meter and 4/10 on the health rating. A study by the Scripps Research Institute had shown that 'burgers, chips and sausages programmed a human brain into craving even more sugar, salt and fat laden food.' Were Martha's school dinners turning her into an addict? With Mary's Meals school dinners were saving lives and changing children's futures for the better but in Scotland it seemed the opposite was happening.

Martha Payne and David Payne

NeverSeconds One primary school pupil's daily dose of school dinners.

FRIDAY 18TH MAY 2012

I totally forgot for half the morning then at lunchtime it came right to my head to tell my friends they are allowed as much salad, bread and fruit as they like. I told them to spread it around the school quickly because no one had gone around the classes and told them. I was a bit nervous to ask but I did ask for more peas!

I chose a Chicken grill which on the old menu was called a chicken burger but it is exactly the same. With it I had chips which means it must be Friday and you can see my extra peas! One of my peas was black, I had a black eyed pea! If you look closely its the one in the middle. I love the sticky gooey icing the school puts on its sponges.

Food-o-meter- 9/10
Mouthfuls- 44, I left the black pea
Courses- main/dessert
Health Rating- 4/10
Price- £2
Pieces of hair- 0

Last year my friends and I started a club, which the school let us run, called Charity Children. We raised money for Mary's Meals. In our first sale we raised £70 in three hours which is enough to feed 7 children school lunches for a WHOLE YEAR! A lot of kids go to school everyday just for the food. Each lunch costs 6p to make.

This is Liberia. It's rice, fish and vegetables. I hope they are eating the meals we paid for.

VEG

Monday 21st May

Our trip to Challenge Gigha was fabulous. Everyone enjoyed racing, we left with a spattering of medals, and Martha was extremely happy with a podium finish even if she hadn't beaten Mum. The phone had remained turned off all day and it wasn't until we sat in the evening sun overlooking the fishing fleet in Tarbert that I switched it back on. The familiar tones for emails, missed calls and messages started and I could see at least an hour's work to get through them all.

I really felt it was important to answer everyone in a reasonable time. Only one in ten emails were from the press now. The rest were from children and parents sharing their stories of their school dinners or of the blogs they were creating, and all were deserving of a reply. I showed Martha a selection of the emails. She answered some herself but I dealt with most, being sure to sign off as Veg's Dad if it was addressed to Veg or Martha's Dad if it was addressed to Martha. I was becoming very used to being called Martha's Dad.

Most of the press enquiries were now coming in from abroad and I was doing radio interviews in Canada, the United States and Australia. The focus was always on the photographs and whether anything had changed in the food on offer. I found it very hard to be positive during these interviews. I always commented on the fact the photographs were a large part of the story and looking through them from this week I was disappointed. Martha had scored her spring rolls with a 3/10 on the food-o-meter despite loving the soup and her health scores averaged only 5/10. Looking through the week's pictures the food was not for Scotland to be proud of nor was it enticing or appetising to me.

Martha and I never discussed her ratings as she wrote her blog and I didn't want to influence her. I wondered if an element of her food-o-meter rating was subconsciously being awarded for looks. Her highest rated meal that week, meatballs, was also the best to look at. The section of her tray was full and the food glistened in the photograph. Now Martha had other school dinners to compare hers with and when her meal was in the same post as a meal from Japan, Taiwan or China the void between the offerings was huge.

Martha was always drawn to the emails from the east and she loved the look of their food. So many items on the plates were completely new to her and despite that she was desperate to try them. The meals sent in were adding an element to the blog that neither Martha nor I had planned. Martha delighted in seeing what had been emailed in and chose the various meals to use herself. Always looking for new foods and new countries, the global nature of her blog was attracting more readers and the number of hits went through one million.

We'd installed a gadget on the page that counted each hit. It looked like a car odometer and you could sit and watch it climb. It was mesmerising to think that each time it clicked on another person was reading the blog. It was lovely when a screen grab appeared in our email showing the moment when her millionth visitor was registered. It was no wonder interview requests kept coming.

Although it was nice to celebrate my daughter's achievements with a wider audience it was also keeping me from my normal work. Lambing was over but with the warmer soil temperatures and increasing daylight I needed to be getting on with planting, and it was not unusual to find me in the polytunnel, mobile in hand and a dibber in the other.

People were taking the time to sit and write comments and take part in NeverSeconds and reading them I was taken by how many people felt it was time for a change.

Martha Payne and David Payne

22 May 2012 03:26

Martha,

As a mommy of a healthy, hearty, hungry little boy, I
want to thank you for making waves in a corrupt food
system. I know your efforts have not gone unnoticed.
I believe that you are helping to create a healthy food
system that will greatly benefit my little boy when he is of
school age and for that I am truly thankful. Keep up the
wonderful work.

Kirsten from North Dakota

It was clear from the comments from America that in places
the problems children were facing were bigger than ours.
Despite being the land of the free it was incredibly hard to get
permission to take photos of school food in America and the
frustration parents were feeling was being expressed in com-
ments and emails. That kept me in tune with the international
reaction to NeverSeconds, but I was deliberately out of touch
with local feelings. There was still no word following on from
my meeting with council officials, but I was pleased that my
local councillor had fixed a date to meet the elected council
leader Mr Roddy McCuish, a Scottish National Party member
from Oban.

Every story has two sides and there was no exception in the
case of Martha's blog. Every supportive tweet, comment and
email we received reassured us that Martha's blog was appreci-
ated and her daily post looked forward to. Martha had stayed
away from commenting upon the stories in the press and had
continued to write simply about 'One primary school pupil's
daily dose of school dinners' as the description at the top of
the blog page said.

But despite the blog's clear labelling there were those that felt
it was an attack on the school dinner staff. Accusations bandied
around on Facebook and so whilst the praise flowed nation-
ally and internationally, locally it did not. I doubted the writers
of these comments were in possession of the full facts but it

was impossible to shake the bewilderment that anyone could believe we would wish to do such a thing. However hurtful some suggestions were, I was able to balance them with the positive comments at the school gates. Cycling friends were starting to dread our next outing as I was channelling my frustration into speed and going far too fast for a good training ride.

When I felt out on a limb, being reminded that there were other people working on the same issues helped. An email from Nick Nairn did just that. Nick was a Scottish chef who made his name being the youngest Scottish chef to win a Michelin Star. I knew of him through a range of his books and television programmes. Back in January Nick had committed to setting up The Menteith Group, a think tank to improve school meals and raise the status of home economics education. With NeverSeconds reopening the school dinner debate, Martha and I were invited to join the day at the Nick Nairn Cook School at Port of Menteith.

The list of attendees was impressive and from a range of companies, local authorities and government departments. It was to be facilitated by Kaye Adams, on whose radio show Malcolm MacFadyen had appeared, and Stephen Jardine, a journalist and founder of Taste Communications. We hadn't taken up any offers to meet anyone yet and it felt right to attend. I was fascinated to hear what the professionals made of Martha's dinners and blog. How important would they feel it was in the great scheme of things? Martha couldn't wait. A chance to meet and cook with a celebrity chef and a day off school. After some of the difficulties, here was a wonderful experience for Martha to have as a reward for her efforts.

WEDNESDAY 23RD MAY 2012

Two, no three, no four fantastic bits of news today!

Whilst I was having my tea my blog went through 1 million hits! I didn't see it but Wrae sent me a photo showing the counter so I haven't missed out, thank you Wrae. When I started writing this I thought only my family and friends would see it so it's amazing so many people have visited and you all care about school food.

My second bit of news is that Dad and I have been invited to a meeting organised by a famous Scottish chef called Nick Nairn. He's invited loads of important people and us to discuss school food and school cooking lessons. I'm really looking forward to meeting him if I can go.

I almost forgot to take a photo today and I had a bite of my burger before I remembered so I turned it around so you can't see it! I had yellow and red peppers, cucumber and roast potatoes. The roast potatoes taste different to the ones at home, My roast potatoes today tasted more like mash. The weather was so nice we were allowed to take our lollies outside.

Food-o-meter- 6/10
Mouthfuls- I lost count when I started licking the lolly
Courses- main/dessert
Health Rating- 4/10
Price- £2
Pieces of hair- 0
Wristband- Orange

Jamie has sent me a photo of a school meal from Yokohama, Japan (33 seconds!)

I only recognise the asparagus, if it is asparagus! Jamie explains,

'I think this one was my favourite, and it had a container of white rice on the side. From the top left and going clockwise, it had:

- pickled daikon radish and sour plum

- steamed sliced okra

- konnyaku jelly (the grey lumpy bits – a high fibre chewy food made from the devil tongue plant. Not much flavour on its own but picks up sauces well) and a chewy rice dumpling thing

- green beans and carrots and garlic

- white fish (mackerel, I think) wrapped in a leaf and steamed

- vegetables and egg cooked with a soy glaze

Taste 8/10
Healthiness 8/10
Price 450 yen (£3.61)'

I recognise the green beans and carrots now! There are so many things I have never tasted.

My last two bits of news? I went to the Dentist and need no fillings again and Mum and Dad came back proud from Parent's Evening at school.

What a day!

VEG

Monday 28th May

"I don't speak German dad!" Martha said over a breakfast of drop pancakes.

"You don't have to. Afra speaks English. She's really funny. You'll like her."

Afra was one of the many German journalists keen to talk to us. Always wanting to support newspapers for children, I'd asked Martha if she would be willing to have a chat on the phone after school.

"But I'll be at Rachel's house."

"Maybe she won't mind if you have quick call there."

NeverSeconds was striking a chord in Germany particularly as school dinners were being introduced in some areas. The debate was certainly beyond tabloid coverage and it was the weekly news magazines that were keen to secure an interview and high-resolution copies of the photographs.

"Can I go on Newsround?"

"Funny you should mention that. They've been in touch asking for an interview with you. Would you like to?"

I knew what the answer would be. All the children watched Newsround every day but were particularly drawn to the Newsround specials available to watch on the website. These specials covered some hard and emotional stories and seemed to grip Martha in particular.

"Would I have to answer questions?"

"You would but I'll be with you. They want to come here and visit you and see the smallholding."

"Will I get make-up?"

"I hope not!"

The Newsround intern who tracked us down was very

reassuring on the phone when I explained we hadn't done any television with Martha but that we would consider Newsround because it was for children. Rebecca and I held the BBC in high regard and felt their ethos was most in tune with ours. Our relationship with the press was becoming more comfortable now. There was less and less interest in the story as it had been told so many times. It was old news and we were happy it was becoming so. We agreed that Newsround could visit in a couple of weeks and that it would mark the end of our involvement in the press. It was something to look forward to and it would be interesting for all of us to see how a film, as it was being called, was made for television. Deals were struck with Polly that if Martha had to have make-up she could as well. Joe on the other hand was promised he would not have to have make-up. Everyone was happy.

Rebecca had grown up holidaying on the Isle of Mull and we'd become regular visitors both to camp and take our stock to the community slaughterhouse. Slaughterhouse trips were family outings. The ferry from Oban wasn't cheap and so if we were going, we made a day of it. A trailer of pigs pulled by a car with bikes or kayaks on top always raised a few eyebrows. They were raised even higher if they knew we were taking the children with us, but the slaughterhouse wasn't an unpleasant place to go for the kids and having them with us helped the animals, who were surrounded by calming familiar faces and voices.

Wednesday was a chance for Rebecca and I to catch up with her parents who were on Mull for the week while the kids were at school. We planned to take our road bikes across on the ferry and cycle the 48 mile Salen, Griben Cliffs, Duart Castle route, meeting Jane and John for a picnic and tea at the castle. We hadn't seen Jane and John since the blog had started and despite our regular phone calls we had much to talk about. It was a fantastically surreal day that epitomises the clashing of cultures as the modern media world rubbed up against Argyll life.

On the ferry crossing we were on the top deck looking for dolphins, porpoises and basking sharks as normal, but I was also speaking to a Hollywood agent who was keen to help us market brand 'Martha and NeverSeconds'. I had exchanged emails with

the agent more for fun and intrigue than anything else. It was clear a lot of thought had been put in at his end. He'd conversed with experts in the field and the consensus was that Martha had the credibility from her Scottish farm background to lead a new movement of peer to peer health education in America. It was felt the launch of the new Disney movie Brave was to be capitalised on. Initial figures were discussed for a cook book written by Martha to start with but hopes were for a television series to follow. I knew the agent was serious. The list of talent that he managed was impressive and even I recognised a string of big names in health and food from America amongst them.

These serious offers were easy to distinguish because payments were offered immediately to Martha and not the other way round. Martha had earning potential and it was guaranteed at $50,000 for the first year with hopes to double it each year for three years. Looking across the sea as the ferry slipped past Duart Castle I wondered who would trade their daughter's childhood for fame and fortune. Martha was no stage school loud and bold girl. She was thoughtful, quiet, a listener and a little shy. Her personality suited her love of writing and nothing could have been more difficult for her than being placed in the spotlight. Hollywood had called the Mull ferry and were told no.

The cycle to picnic at the foot of Ben More, Mull's only Munro, was leisurely and with quiet roads Rebecca and I could chat the whole way. Jane and John were waiting for us with a fabulous spread, far more than was wise to eat with big hills and more miles ahead. Sat on a blanket in the sun I was explaining to John some of the offers that had come in.

"We've been invited to Taiwan, Japan and the USA all flights paid for. We've had an offer of £20,000 for the website and with the hits coming to the website we could earn an estimated $35,000 by putting ads on it."

"You wouldn't though, would you?"

"No. It would change everything if adverts appeared. I don't think it would have the same credibility if it was seen that a nine year old was trying to make money. Other kids would stop supporting it. It wouldn't be special anymore."

Technically it's very easy to put adverts on your blog. Five minutes on the BlogSpot web interface and it would be done.

"I've had emails asking how to support Mary's Meals and Martha is getting some money from magazines that she'd like to donate. Maybe we should set up a JustGiving page for donations to Mary's Meals. That way no funds come to us at all and there can be no doubt it all goes to Mary's Meals."

John's knowledge of Mary's Meals through his talks was huge and he was able to explain that £7000 would build and equip a kitchen for a school in Malawi. It seemed a great total to aim for.

"We'll have to go and see it if we raise all the money," Rebecca said as we slowly climbed up the side of Glen Gorm, back on the bikes.

"Och no. It's too far and too expensive."

Rebecca, Jane and John had all visited Africa before. John and Jane as volunteers 40 years ago and Rebecca more recently on a medical elective to Uganda in 1997.

"It'll make a huge impression on the kids. They'll love it."

It was true the kids were great at making friends and on that level it would be fun for them.

A Malawian school could have 2000 primary children or more and would be larger than the Lochgilphead Joint Campus. How the kids would react to the numbers of children, the long walks to school and the poverty the children lived in I wasn't sure. With the innate sense of natural justice children have I knew Martha would struggle to understand how it could be so unfair and in turn she would force me to confront these issues so I could explain them to her. Somehow I lived every day with the knowledge that it wasn't fair or right, and didn't feel embarrassed about doing so. It was easier to ignore than to confront but I didn't want to teach that to my children.

Duart Castle tea rooms was a welcome stop. Between mouthfuls of home baked scone I was being interviewed by Der Spiegel news magazine from Germany. With a circulation of one million copies and its massive online presence it was no wonder the interview was in depth. Pushed hard on the causes of poor meals in Scotland, I needed to repeat that I was not an expert on the provision of school food. Scotland did have a food culture but when you were more famous as a nation for deep fried Mars bars than fine seafood, beef and soft fruits, then there was work to be done. Martha's blog was not helping to change the image

of a country obsessed with fast food.

"Do the council realise that Martha is blogging?"

"Yes. I asked for permission from the school before she started to photograph and write about her dinners."

"So the council know she is sharing the dinner and yet they feed her that? Interesting. In Germany how we feed our children is important. It is a measure of the country, no?"

There was no answer I could give.

The ferry back to Oban was crowded with day trippers like ourselves. Up on deck our thin cycling clothes weren't much protection from the sea breeze. Cuddling up for warmth I whispered to Rebecca, "People think this is a dream come true you know. I think it's a bit of a nightmare."

Before she could answer the phone rang again.

"Hello, is that Mr Payne. I'm calling from Nine Lives Media and we're making a Channel 4 Dispatches documentary on school food because of Martha's blog and we'd like you to be involved..."

MONDAY 28TH MAY 2012

We were practicing Olympic athletic events at school this morning in PE so I was very hungry come lunchtime and it didn't help that my year were second last in the queue! My sister and I were a bit nervous that we would get into trouble asking for fruit with our lunch today so Dad printed off an email from the council and my sister put it in her school bag. I had to ask for fruit and they were unsure but when they checked it was ok.

Today's Shepherd's Pie was really nice. The mash on top was really creamy and the mince was in lovely gravy. I wonder where their meat comes from. The salad was lovely and crunchy. The cake looked really difficult to serve because the icing was so sticky. I saved my melon until last and it was a great way to end my lunch.

Food-o-meter- 9/10
Mouthfuls- 32
Courses- main/dessert
Health Rating- 7/10
Price- £2
Pieces of hair- 0
Wristband- Yellow

Miranda from the Unites States of America (1 second! Would have been longer but Miranda didn't mention where she is in the USA) has sent this photo of her lunch. She says its bigger because she is at High School for grade 9-12.

Miranda says it's an example of the worst food she gets at school because the spaghetti has a dye in that stains and that the milk is very sweet. She enjoys the salad, as long as it has a dressing and says 'the gummies, not much to say about them, they are simply gummies. Good gummies at that :-)'

Martha Payne and David Payne

Food-O-Meter: 5/10
Mouthfuls: 51
Courses: All one course. We go up and choose what we
want, and it is put on our (flimsy styrofoam) platter.
Generally, we get one main course (the spaghetti) with
a side course (the bread), a drink (the cocoa milk) and 2
mini-sides (the salad and gummy candies). Anything else is
charged extra.
Health rating: 3/10
Price: 1.42 quid (that's 2.25 american dollars. sorry
I could not put the pound sign, my keyboard is not
international)
Pieces of hair: 0
Veggies: I took a salad, that's about 5/10, 14 mouthfuls.

Miranda I have no idea what gummies are but I am glad you
like them! What is very different is I think you bin your
tray and fork where as ours get washed. Do you recycle
them?

It's sports day tomorrow and I hope tomorrow's lunch is
as good as today's as we are racing all afternoon!

VEG

Sunday 3rd June

The road to Campbeltown, which sits at the bottom of the Mull
of Kintyre, takes about an hour from Lochgilphead and twists
and winds through Tarbert then to the shore and long beaches
at Machrihanish. The whole family were travelling down for the
annual Mull of Kintyre Half Marathon, which involved running
along the very beach we could see stretching out for miles ahead
of us. Rebecca was running the 10km and the kids were looking
forward to the children's races. It was a sunny day and I joined
my fellow runners and headed to the start. Not being a fast
runner I made sure I wasn't blocking the elite runners when I
was jostled from the back.

"You NeverSecond's Dad?"

"Aye," I said nervously.

The runner grabbed my hand.

"You should be so proud. What are the council doing, feeding
our kids that crap? They're throwing away our next generation's
health. Good on you. Stick it to them."

Before I could explain it was a writing project the hooter
sounded and we were off. I tried desperately to catch up with
him to continue the chat but he was away weaving in the crowd.
My training for the race had imprinted on me the need to pace
myself. I knew the first seven miles would feel easy. The atmos-
phere in the town was fabulous and with folk cheering I would
be buoyed along. The next three miles including running on the
beach would be hard. Tiredness would be creeping into the legs
and the soft sand would suck energy. The last three miles into
the wind and uphill before dropping into the town to the finish
was where I would need to rely on mental toughness. It's not
my speciality and true to form at the ten mile mark my whole

body was telling me to quit. I was telling myself I'd gone too hard too early and that I was blown. I was lining the excuses up in my mind to tell club mates at the finish when I saw the runner from the start ahead of me. I could catch him. I had to catch him. I picked up the cadence concentrating on the rhythm of my feet hitting the pavement. I pulled alongside.

"It's... it's... it's a writing project," I managed to say as we ran side by side. Mile eleven of a half marathon at my level of fitness is not the place for an in depth discussion. It wasn't for him either.

"Official complaint. Can't... ignore... you... then." He was slowing, "GO!" he shouted.

My mind was distracted now. I had things to get angry about. Council staff on national radio attacking Martha for bringing to light the deficiencies in their service. A meeting in which we had agreed to differ and move forward with a press release only for the council to renaig. They were deaf to our concerns and attempts to be proactive with them. My fellow runner was right. I needed to complain. I started to sketch out in my mind the complaint letter. I was completely distracted from the race but as the anger in me rose my pace picked up. I was flying and ahead the line loomed and I crossed it with a time of 1 hour 45 minutes and a letter in my head. I had made it and had just enough time to walk over and see Martha in the girls' race.

Martha loves running almost as much as she loves winning and I could see her at the start line, haired tied back, looking along the line of racers working out who was the competition. As the starter called them to the line she was squeezed into the second row of runners and a moment of panic crossed her face. She looked to the crowd and I could see her mum give her a nod. Rebecca spent so much time working and away from the family that you would think that her relationship with the kids would suffer. I saw the strain on Rebecca's face some days when she returned home from the hospital. She might have been hours managing a road crash victim waiting for the Retrieval Service to helicopter in consultants from Glasgow or supporting a family whose loved one had passed away in the hospital. However hard it had been, she left it outside our home so when she walked in and Polly and Martha shouted 'Mummy' she was

there, arms open, strain gone and smiling as they hugged. That nod from Mum settled Martha and once the hooter went she was off. Martha ran with no awkwardness and was balanced as she accelerated hard from the start, too hard, and had to stop for a breath.

"Pace it Martha," I shouted, "go steady!"

She saw me in the crowd, smiled and set off again. She sneaked back through the field heading for the front. She hadn't given in and crossed the line to a deserved cheer for third place. I wasn't going to give in either and once home I used Argyll and Bute's online form to submit my race-crafted complaint.

'Our complaint comprises of 5 elements.

1) On Radio Scotland Malcolm MacFadyen blamed our daughter for the plate of food she had. In truth she chose one of the 4 set menus and was served a full portion of that meal. She could not have had any more food under the rules in use then.

2) On Radio Scotland Malcolm MacFadyen inferred blame lies with us as parents.

3) Jayne Murphy on You and Yours blamed Martha. Martha chose one of the 4 set menus and was served a full portion of that meal. She could not have had any more food under the rules in use then.

4) The press release given to the BBC was erroneous in its claim that there was unlimited bread and salad available to children.

5) As Martha chose a full meal of the menu, which resulted in the food she blogged on the 8th May, we are complaining that the lunches were of an unacceptable quantity and quality.'

I received an acknowledgement and it was just a case of waiting the twenty days allowed. Martha noticed I'd finished typing.

"What were you doing, Dad?"

"I was writing a complaint letter to the council about what they said on the radio and your dinners."

"Oh. What do they do about it?"

"They have to look at what they said and decide if it was

right or wrong."

"But it was wrong. I know that. I eat there every day, they don't."

She had a good point.

"Can I make my JustGiving page now?"

"Of course."

We settled down. JustGiving's website allowed visitors to make donations to charities via individuals that supported them. Like the sponsorship forms I used to cajole family to sign, but available to the world. We already had an account with JustGiving from various donations we'd previously made and the process of designing Martha's NeverSeconds page was swift. Grandpa John had sent over an email with the info on Mary's Meals and Martha used her word processing skills to copy and paste it into the 'story' section of the page along with her writing.

"I am going to use the £50 from Der Spiegel to start it with."

Entering the donation for £50 I hoped the money would turn up. It seemed to be the going rate and whilst Der Spiegel had offered it as a matter of course most magazines and papers did not.

"That will provide a school dinner for nearly 5 children for a year."

"You should ask them for exactly 5 children."

Martha opened the calculator on the laptop. "That's £53.50."

That's what we did from then on. I found it easy to ask for a donation to the JustGiving page and companies had no issue with doing so and seemed impressed that £10.70 could do so much.

"Are you still enjoying blogging?" I asked, hoping she was. She was so sheltered from the global debate and with her brother and sister also busy it wasn't much discussed at home. She knew it was her choice and some evenings I didn't remind her to blog, waiting instead for her to pick up the laptop if she wished.

"You think I should stop don't you?"

It had been easy to take media decisions on Martha's behalf so far. In years to come she might regret the missed opportunities to travel. I would have loved to have joined her in Japan but she could travel later in life. Deciding to stop blogging was

going to have to be a decision for Martha.

"I don't want to say you should or shouldn't," I said.

"But you think I should?"

The news had moved on and if she stopped now those that thought it was some kind of orchestrated publicity stunt would take it as a sign.

"If you enjoying taking the photos and writing then do it. It's a great project and I think you can take it to the end of term. It's only three weeks until the holidays and no school dinners then."

"No school dinners but camping food!"

She was already looking forward to our summer trips in the trailer tent and so was I.

MONDAY 11TH JUNE 2012

Drawn

I absolutely totally forgot my camera again today. Well I didn't totally forget it because I got it into my school bag but not from my school bag to the lunch hall. I was so keen to eat I dashed out of my class leaving the camera behind. So today I have drawn my lunch for you on the computer!

In case you can't tell I had carrot and coriander soup to start which is still my favourite and I would pick it over chocolate cake any day. The soup was so hot after one mouthful I nearly burnt my mouth so I had it after my main. I chose an omelette over the sausages because I haven't had it for a while. It was really nice and tasted of cheese. With it I had roast potatoes which are never crunchy, radishes, pineapple and cucumber. The radishes were crunchy and spicey! I ate absolutely everything but I was too full for fruit.

Food-o-meter- 9/10
Mouthfuls- thirty something
Courses- starter/main
Health Rating- 8/10
Price- £2
Pieces of hair- 0
Wristband- Yellow

Mary's Meal Total-170 children fed for a year or 25% of a kitchen. Thank you!

I am getting excited about meeting all the people with Nick Nairn this week to talk about food. It's going to be awesome!

VEG

Monday 11th June

"So silly of me," Martha berated herself for forgetting to take a photo. "I left it in my bag and just pure forgot."

"So will you blog?" I should have known the answer because Martha was grabbing the laptop from where it was charging and heading to the sofa.

"I'm going to draw my lunch instead."

Her determined voice said it all. Showing her how to open the paint software in the computer I saw her grimace as she shuffled along the sofa.

"My wrist's sore, Dad. I tripped at athletics club and landed on it."

Her mum was on call and in the hospital so we agreed to wait until she came home to see what she made of it.

Her picture was coming together and with her description it was a fair representation of her lunch but clearly a photo was better. She had been sent many drawings of food from children who were not allowed to take cameras into school but Martha hadn't chosen to use any on the blog. Even the best drawings lacked the impact that a photo made. A good photograph gave the blog readers so much. From the shine of the gravy to the crumbs of the cakes there were clues from a photograph to say how the food would taste. That dull green of overcooked broccoli alongside the vibrantly coloured jelly was a contrast few colouring pen sets could match.

"Only one more lunch," she smiled, "before we visit Granny and Grandpa and then Nick Nairn's!"

It wasn't clear which was the most exciting to her. With three children, adventures involving just one don't come along often and I was really pleased to be spending some time with

Martha. All of the kids are most chatty in the front of the car and on even short journeys the conversations could be insightful. Joe often took the time to describe his latest creations in MineCraft, an online game, in which he and his friends co-operated via the internet and built houses and dens in a virtual world. MineCraft seemed to have its own language and it was hard to understand exactly what was meant by 'mods' and 'slave servers'. Joe had taken Martha's blog in his stride. At no point had he ever expressed any signs of jealousy towards the attention she was receiving. I'm not sure he understood why she enjoyed writing and the feeling was mutual, as Martha had little time for MineCraft.

"We'll go tomorrow evening and stay the night at Granny's. I've got to get to the Cook School for the morning but Granny and Grandpa will bring you over for lunch."

"I won't be on my own will I?"

Her strong writing style wasn't fully matched with confidence in new situations and I reassured her she would always be with one of the family. I knew Granny and Grandpa would keep her right. Through the weeks they had kept buying the articles she was featured in and helped me stay on top of what was being said with regular emails. Going to the Cook School at Port of Menteith had been discussed with them and the rest of the family before we had accepted the invitation. We'd agreed to a photographer coming from the Daily Record to take some photos of Nick and Martha. It was a case of falling back again on the principle that whatever Martha did should have a clear benefit for others. Feeling as we did that school dinners needed to be improved not just for Martha but for the next generation of Scottish children, we agreed. The chef and the schoolgirl both passionate about school dinners was a story we were happy to support. I had already asked the school if it was ok for Martha to wear her school uniform in the photos. I wasn't even sure if I needed to ask but it seemed the right thing to do. Some consternation was caused and it was a while before it was agreed. Martha was proud of her school and wearing the uniform was a way for her to express it.

The following morning was spent at the hospital getting Martha's sore wrist x-rayed. The growth plate at the end of her

radius had broken away and a cast was needed, a stookie as it's called in Scotland. Martha started off loving the idea of a stookie but the reality was soon to hit.

"I can't wash. That's cool!"

"Yeah brilliant. You're meeting Nick and you'll be a bit whiffy." She knew I was joking.

"Nick can sign it tomorrow."

The nurse pointed out that it was a temporary cast until the swelling went down and she wouldn't have the proper cast until after she had met him. Martha was not impressed. Her blog that night was clear. Her school dinner had cheered her up. She heaped praise on the macaroni cheese and described sucking jelly through her teeth. With a solid 10/10 on the food-o-meter it was as good as it got and after a morning of disappointments her dinner had put a smile on her face.

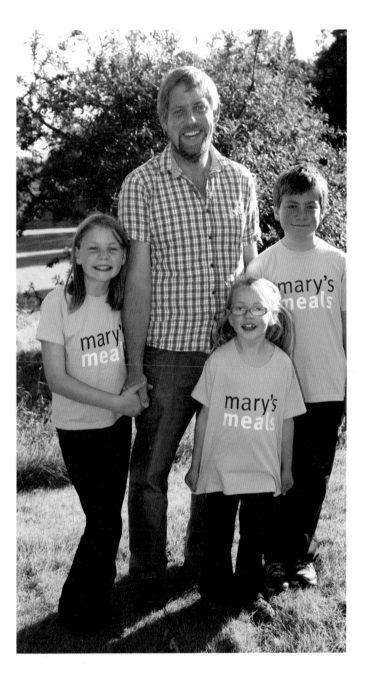

TUESDAY 12TH JUNE 2012

Broken!

Unfortunately I have to choose my lunches differently now because I have only 1 hand to eat with. Last night at athletics club in the first race I tripped and fell on my hand. It was still sore this morning so I went to hospital and ended up with a stookie on my wrist. 'Stookie' is our Scots word for a plaster cast. My dinners will have to be easy to eat for the next few weeks. My friends are really helpful and they helped me carry my tray at dinner.

Lunch was really nice today and it helped cheer me up. Macaroni Cheese at school is so creamy and it's nice to have it with the crunchy radishes and peppers. You don't have to have mash with the macaroni but they offered me some and I took it as I always have mash if it's offered. We don't get jelly often, maybe about twice in every 4 weeks, and I like to put it on my spoon and suck it through my teeth. It's so slippy it doesn't really make a noise so I don't upset my friends!

Food-o-meter- 10/10
Mouthfuls- 37
Courses- main/dessert
Health Rating- 5/10
Price- £2
Pieces of hair- 0
Ease of eating with wrist in stookie- 9/10
Wristband- Yellow

Mary's Meal Total-180 children fed for a year or 25.8% of a kitchen. Thank you!

VEG

Wednesday 13th June

The dreaded red 'STOP' light on the dashboard lit up less than a mile from Granny's house and the inevitable cruise to a stand-still would no doubt be followed by an equally inevitable large bill for a repair. I was very grateful to the breakdown company and the garage that got me into a courtesy car and away so I was only an hour late to the Cook School at Port of Menteith. Signs led me to a modern building tucked away in the beautiful Stirlingshire countryside at the foothills of the Trossachs.

My cooking skills were taught to me by my mum, who always produced the hearty meals loved by teenage boys despite working fulltime. Going to a cookery school was a new experience and, unsure what was awaiting me, I paused and took a deep breath. Inside I was greeted by our contact Sophie, who led me through the shop to the demonstration kitchen. Behind the counter Nick Nairn and Stephen Jardine were facilitating the discussion and some of Martha's photos were projected onto the wall. A quick introduction from Nick led to the inevitable red flush and I took my place amongst the 30 or so delegates and listened. My credentials for being there were probably the weakest in the room. Martha's Dad and smallholder didn't quite stand up against a Scottish Government Inspector or a Professor of Nutrition and listening was to be the order of the day.

It was fascinating. Nick had a range of ingredients in front of him all costing the £1.05 average that is spent on ingredients in a Scottish school dinner and demonstrated how a simple and tasty meal could be cooked quickly and healthily. I was pleased because the couscous and pasta dishes were a staple of my home cooking. Discussions sparked off about the use of salt in soup and bread rolls. Salt has such a negative effect on health that

even a roll could sway the balance of a meal from good to bad. A range of fresh vegetables were available to use in the dishes and it was debated as to whether frozen had better nutrients.

Then it was our turn to pair off and cook. I could understand why Nick was a firm believer in cooking as a great way to start conversations and bring strangers together. Soon I was chatting away to Carina Contini, owner of The Scottish Café and Centotre restaurant in Edinburgh and also a campaigner trying to improve school meals in her children's primary school. The knife flashed as she made short work of the onion and garlic in front of her before using the knife to scoop them up and flick them into a pot. Out skilled, I bumbled along next to her grateful for her warmth and kindness to Martha and her blog. At every workstation there were smiles and the clink of the pans on the hobs was the only sound to interrupt the buzz of conversation. I saw Martha with her grandparents chatting to Nick and Stephen. Martha was smiling and showing off her stookie happily. If she was feeling shy it wasn't showing and she was the more relaxed of the two of us. We all had prison trays like Martha's with compartments to eat from and as we passed from the kitchen Sophie took a photo and Martha cast her eye over them looking for the day's winner.

As we sat down to eat Nick and Martha took to the kitchen to cook. The photographer joined them and along with Grandpa took some snaps. Excited after her lesson Martha joined me to enjoy her lunch.

"It was brilliant, Dad! Nick made huge flames but he didn't burn the food. Can you do that?"

"Not intentionally," I replied as Martha tucked into her lunch.

She was really enjoying the experience as were Granny and Grandpa who had managed to find a fellow Mary's Meals supporter amongst the guests. Martha's JustGiving page was being well received and the donations added up to almost £2000. She was keen to tell anyone that would listen that she was almost a third of the way to her target. Before leaving Martha chose her meal of the day and Professor of Human Nutrition Mike Lean took the honours, giving Nick the chance to joke about being out cooked!

Kaye Adams, who had interviewed Malcolm MacFadyen from Argyll and Bute council on her radio programme, was facilitating the afternoon. Keeping tabs on a room of eager to speak individuals and keeping the conversation on track wasn't easy but Kaye managed to steer the room from topic to topic. The Schools (Health Promotion and Nutrition) (Scotland) Act 2007 was being held up as an example that other countries were looking to follow. Examples of good practice were shared along with case studies of primary school engagement in the Soil Association's Food for Life scheme. It was blisteringly good stuff and the theme linking all the best examples was that behind each was a brilliant, passionate individual inspiring those around them to deliver an excellent service. It was impossible however to forget the dinners Martha was blogging. They did not fit this picture of excellence painted in the discussion. They showed the opposite end of the scale, where the applauded Scottish Government Act was being used as a minimum standard to meet rather than a springboard to launch from. I had to wonder how many other children's meals across Scotland were like Martha's. I added to the discussion.

"I feel the dining hall should be another classroom. The lesson everyday should be the best lesson we can give the kids in food and healthy eating. The dining hall is often at the heart of the school and food can be at the heart of many subjects from maths to English."

Teachers didn't shy away from teaching the hard lessons in the curriculum and I didn't see why we should give up on the hard lessons of food. The Scottish nation's poor health was continuing to decline. Whatever way it was being tackled clearly wasn't working. Changing how school dinners were delivered and how we taught our next generation to eat should have been the new priorities. It really was time that Scotland developed a food culture to be proud of and left deep fried Mars bars behind. It didn't matter how healthy they made the pizzas, hot dogs and burgers in school. If schools continued to feed them to our children we would be giving them the stamp of approval and we shouldn't be surprised when pizzas, hot dogs and burgers became part of their diet for life.

I was taken by Fife Diet's Mike Small's stated aim that all

children leaving primary school should be able to make a pot of soup. It was shocking to hear that primary aged children could leave the school at lunchtime to eat junk food in town. I thought children should be encouraged to photograph their dinners and to write about them. Martha had thought more about what she ate since starting NeverSeconds than ever before, but consternation flared in the room at the idea of children blogging.

"It could be abused."

"How could we police it?"

How about school's also publishing, tweeting or blogging a photo each day? Parents could compare their child's photos and school photos. Whilst the Soil Association's scheme aimed to make changes it relied upon the local authorities to engage with it, and those like Argyll and Bute who were happy with their standard of dinner simply ignored it. An award scheme in which children were the motivators and change makers could not be disregarded. Free lunches to all Scottish Primary school children and no option to leave the grounds. Each child's choice of lunch could influence whether the school gained the next tier or flag of the award structure. Small steps to start with, leading to giant bounds as the children rose through the school. Visiting a local food producer, blogging for a week, visiting the kitchens to learn a recipe to cook at home, growing vegetables and keeping chickens; all these elements could combine to launch our children into their adult life with healthy habits and the ability to make informed choices about food. It had been an inspiring day and making our farewells before the long drive home I was heartened that there was an aspiration for change. The hard part would be making it a reality.

WEDNESDAY 13TH JUNE 2012

A different day.

I joined Nick Nairn at his cookery school for lunch today.
Lots of adults who care about school dinners were there
and they all cooked a school lunch and photographed it.
I chose the one I liked best. Everyone was really friendly
and I enjoyed speaking to them. Nick showed me how to
make lunch and it was quick and really tasty and cost the
same as my lunches. I ate it all.

Unluckily our car broke down today and my arm is sore and
we are late home so I will post more tomorrow. Today has
been a new and great experience.

VEG

Thursday 14th June

Big hands and small phones don't work and I was struggling to send Rebecca a text.

"Daily Record. Nice pic. Dodgy headline. Time to fire the dinner ladies."

"What?" she texted a reply.

"Headline over flame cooking photo. Time to fire the dinner ladies. Not funny"

"Bad joke."

I'd grabbed a copy of the paper at the garage and was sat in the car texting with the article on my lap in front of me. I'd been led to believe that feelings were already running high in the kitchens. I was at a loss as to why. Martha only ever spoke in the nicest terms of the lunchtime staff and never a cross word was directed to her from them. Of course Martha's blog was throwing light on the dinners they were providing but Martha understood that the decisions on menus and quantities were not taken by the dinner ladies but by their managers.

The absolute ban on all council employees discussing the matter with us or the press was to the detriment of all. The council had repeatedly gone on national radio to defend their school dinner service stating that NeverSeconds reflected only one child's choice but had failed to provide any other examples. Given half a chance to chat with Martha's teacher I would have been suggesting that her whole class blogged their lunches for a week. NeverSeconds could have published the whole classes writing and photographs. As a project embracing the new Curriculum for Excellence in Scotland it would have been magnificent. The positive spin the council communications team could have put out celebrating Martha's inspiring

teacher and their school which was able to respond quickly to join in on a fabulous worldwide project would have been PR gold. These ideas would need a spirit of cooperation, one I had already shown by arranging a meeting, but instead of finding an imaginative solution that could triumph the wider range of school dinners they had bought the dinner ladies flowers.

Martha was out of sorts coming out of school. Head down she shuffled over the playground to where I was waiting.

"Can we just go now?" She was avoiding making eye contact with everyone, her friends, the other kids and me. She set off around the corner to the car while I waited on Polly. As we drove out of the school, crossing the line that marked the end of the school grounds, Martha dissolved. It was a while before she could talk and through sobs she tried to explain.

"I was taken out of class this morning by the head teacher and told to stop taking photos. Everyone in school knows."

I could hear the pain and humiliation her voice.

"Were you told why?"

"Because of a stupid newspaper headline. Mrs Stankey said she knew it wasn't my fault."

"Oh love."

Martha looked at me for the first time and I could see the redness circling each eye from the tears.

"Because she banned me everyone thinks I was doing something wrong now. I wasn't was I?"

"No Martha you weren't. I'll phone when we get home."

The rest of the journey home was in silence. It seemed the duty of care owed to Martha by her school and the council had been thrown out of the window. She had been told the news in the middle of the morning. No attempt had been made from the school or from the council to contact me and there was no letter in Martha's bag to explain. It struck me as a cowardly way to behave. To drag a nine year old into the office on her own would leave any child bewildered, upset and scared. To do so without good reason and without consulting her parents was a dereliction of their duty of care to her and to us. The pressure from the council headquarters on the head teacher must have been huge for her to do such a thing and it's thanks to the good relationship the head maintains with her children that more

damage to Martha wasn't done.

"Have some electronic time kids," I said as we arrived home.

I checked both my landline and mobile phone. No messages or missed calls on either. I listened to my messages to double check and examined my emails. I was incredulous. The spinelessness of the council to choose to convey its decision through a nine year old should have surprised me but it didn't.

"Can I speak to the communications team please?" I asked the switchboard operator at Argyll and Bute Council headquarters. I took deep breaths waiting to be connected.

"Hello?"

"Hi. It's David Payne here. Is that Lindsey? I think we spoke last time I called the council."

"Yes it's Lindsey. Hello Mr Payne."

"Lindsey, did you know they've banned Martha from taking photos?"

"Er no. We've not been told anything."

"Well I'm not sure but I think this might blow up again. It could be a long few days for us both. I'm sorry."

"I'll find out what's going on and get someone to call you."

"Thanks."

Putting the phone down I wondered if it really might flare up again. I sat down and read her last entries. A generous 10/10 on the food-o-meter for the last meal. Only 5/10 for health but it was macaroni cheese and jelly. Her post about meeting Nick Nairn was entirely uncontroversial. Anyone reading the blog would be confused as to why it was banned. It wasn't a tirade written against individuals aiming to cause upset, it was simply her daily dose of school dinners. The phone rang and I picked it up.

"Hello?"

"Mr Payne, it's Cleland Sneddon here. I'm Director of Community Services and it was my decision to ban the photographs."

So started the most shocking and offensive phone call I have ever received. It wasn't a conversation because that would imply he listened to what I had to say. When I spoke he laughed down the phone at me and continued to do so after I pointed out how rude and offensive he was being. He went on to say that if

another word was written on the blog the council would have to defend itself against these unwarranted attacks. I felt like I was being threatened. His words seemed deliberately chosen to be hurtful. He sounded practiced in the language of a playground bully and he weaved intimidation and inferences on Martha's honesty into a rant that lasted 28 minutes 16 seconds. Here was one of Argyll and Bute Council's most senior employees showing his true colours. It was clear to me that the man whose job was to look after the education of our children, provide services for the elderly and most vulnerable people in our community, was reacting to a joke headline in a tabloid newspaper by threatening to destroy the integrity of a nine-year-old girl.

I replaced the phone in its cradle. Those 28 minutes and 16 seconds were to change everything. If I had recorded the conversation I would have handed it to the police. Whilst I had no doubt he would carry out his threats I knew that Martha was not at fault, and to give in to the playground bully was not an example I was about to set to Joe, Martha, Polly or any of the thousands of children that read the blog.

"Hey Martha," I carried the laptop over to her. "What are you going to say today?"

I opened up the page for a new post.

"Do you mind if I add a bit on the bottom after you, something about what happened today?" I added.

"OK Dad. But I've got to read it first."

As Martha started to write her final entry I began an email conversation with Grandpa John. I wanted to name and shame Cleland Sneddon in my part of the post but John's advice was clearly not to do so. Starting an argument with an individual would detract from the real issue, which was the council's decision to ban Martha taking photos. Even after broken promises of joint press releases we hadn't let the behaviour of the council become the debate and using the proper complaint channels was more appropriate than fighting through the press.

I finished drafting my part of the post and showed it to Martha.

"It's like mine, Dad," she said, turning the laptop so I could read her entry. "I've not written much."

Her entry was perfect. It didn't blame, it simply reported

the facts and how she felt. It was like every other post she had written.

Everyone needs a little luck and ours was provided in the form of our good friends Steve and Hazel. Both triathletes, they heard the news of the ban from Rebecca in between lengths at the triathlon club training night. I'd shared the ups and downs of the blog with them both over cycles and runs, and beyond the family no one was more informed than they were. Hazel works alongside Rebecca in the Accident & Emergency section of the hospital and Steve is a senior manager in the NHS. When they appeared at the door with Rebecca after swimming they brought not just a bottle of wine but calm and analytical minds.

The tone and content of my phone call from Cleland Sneddon came as no surprise to them. Although I hadn't heard of him before it seemed his response was very much in character. Twitter and Facebook were lighting up with news of the ban and emails and alerts were beginning to build. Journalists I had not spoken to for weeks were now trying to get in contact again and the flurry of interest a month before was starting to look like a warm up to the impending main event. I was up and down answering the phone, and during one call I stopped in my tracks and waved to Rebecca, Steve and Hazel for silence.

"The Today Programme?" I questioned, unable to quite to believe it.

The Today Programme was the news and current affairs morning radio programme on BBC Radio 4. It was listened to by over 6 million and was the first choice of politicians, so if you weren't news before appearing on the programme you were afterwards. I looked for reassurance to Rebecca. She nodded back her agreement and it was settled. I would be giving a live telephone interview at 7.20 the following morning, a Friday. I was shaky sitting down.

"Blimey. Better get our thinking caps on," I announced.

Smallholding had been my only job for years and I was far removed from the corporate world that Steve operated in. His insight into the behaviour of the council confirmed my feelings that the appalling decision to ban Martha's photographs had come as a result of the long string of management failures that had characterised the story so far. For the next half hour

we bandied ideas and phrases around. The tone we settled upon was to express disappointment in the decision, not to mention individuals, to support the school and make it clear it was a council decision. When we hit upon the right line I wrote it down in a box on a sheet of A4. With twelve boxes to a side we managed to fill three sheets and I then set about grouping the boxes into topics. I was left with was a set of crib sheets that weren't to leave my pocket for the next 36 hours.

It was a sleepless night. The council had already shown how low it could go. But whilst they thought they had carried out their latest act of intimidation towards Martha in private, they had in fact been witnessed by hundreds of thousands of people who were about to stand up and be counted. The protective arms of the internet hadn't been able to prevent Martha's fall but they were about to cushion her landing.

THURSDAY 14TH JUNE 2012

Goodbye.

This morning in maths I got taken out of class by my head teacher and taken to her office. I was told that I could not take any more photos of my school dinners because of a headline in a newspaper today.

I only write my blog not newspapers and I am sad I am no longer allowed to take photos. I will miss sharing and rating my school dinners and I'll miss seeing the dinners you send me too. I don't think I will be able to finish raising enough money for a kitchen for Mary's Meals either.

Goodbye,

VEG

Hi,

Veg's Dad, Dave, here. I felt it's important to add a few bits of info to the blog tonight. Martha's school have been brilliant and supportive from the beginning and I'd like to thank them all. I contacted Argyll and Bute Council when Martha told me what happened at school today and they told me it was their decision to ban Martha's photography.

It is a shame that a blog that today went through 2 million hits, which has inspired debates at home and abroad and raised nearly £2000 for charity is forced to end.

Dave Payne
neverseconds@gmail.com

Friday 15th June

There was no need to set an alarm. I watched the time on the clock tick away until 6.30am and slipped out of bed. I'd normally switch the kitchen radio onto the Today programme as I made my coffee but I hesitated. The voices of Evan Davis and Sarah Montague who were presenting the show were familiar to me but to listen to them in the run up to my interview would have shredded my already sleep deprived nerves. The temptation to dip into emails, the blog or twitter was huge. There would be messages of support and journalists all needing replies. In the end I was glad I hadn't, as I would have been overwhelmed. Unbeknown to me the blog counter couldn't keep up and there were several hundred comments awaiting moderation. On twitter #NeverSeconds was trending at number three in the world and it was soon to be joined by Martha, Mary's Meals and Argyll and Bute in the top ten.

Ten minutes before the interview the crib sheet came out. I added a separate column of items to avoid discussing. The phone rang, it was to be Sarah Montague interviewing and I waited, listening to the programme through the telephone. At 7.24am we were off.

Sarah: "Last month a nine year old school girl started a blog about her school dinners. Martha Payne took photographs, rated the meals and commented on them. It was a huge success with her website taking a million hits in just the first month. Even Jamie Oliver called it a shocking but inspirational blog. Now though the school has told her she can no longer take photos of the dinners making it hard for her to continue the blog. In fact the last post yesterday said goodbye. Her father

David Payne joins us now. Good Morning."

Me: "Good Morning."

Sarah: "Initially it seems the reaction of the school was very positive to what Martha was doing. So what happened?"

Me: "I think the school is continuing to be very positive. There was an unfortunate headline given to a photograph in a newspaper which caused the council to take the decision above school level that Martha was no longer to be allowed to take photographs."

Sarah: "So it was the council's decision to ban the photographs."

Me: "It was. It was above the school. The school have been very supportive and the reason Martha started a writing project and writing about food was the inspiration from a teacher to write in the style of a journalist."

Sarah: "We should say we did actually approach the council to see if they could give us a statement or some comment but they, it's Argyll and Bute Council, but they weren't able to provide us with one for whatever reason. The headline in the newspaper was though about firing school dinners. Was that what Martha was, I mean... I mean look she's nine, but is that what she was aware might happen as a result of her blogs?"

Me: "No. I don't think she was and none of us were. The project started because she was enjoying writing and because she wanted to be a journalist. A blog has the element of publishing, about putting something out there in the style of a newspaper and we honestly thought it would be family and aunts and uncles and grannies and grandpas that would read it. We didn't expect [Sarah chuckles] there to be headlines such as that appearing in the press no."

Sarah: "Nor I suppose for 2 million people to have seen it since she started doing it."

Me: "Indeed. The numbers are staggering really and people talk about things going viral but until it happens you don't really understand how it does and I still don't."

Sarah: "And we should say it wasn't all critical, some of her posts and the photographs don't look bad at all."

Me: "Oh indeed. The last photograph of a meal at school that she blogged she gave ten out of ten. She couldn't have awarded

it a higher mark and she enjoys the atmosphere in the school dining hall. She enjoys meeting the staff there and everyone has been very kind to her and absolutely no complaints from us."

Sarah: "So that's it for the blog? I suspect we are going to hear from her again in some form."

Me: "Anyone knowing Martha will know she'll make her own mind up. She's enjoyed writing but the photos tell so much of it and it makes it a focal point for her to write about but I'd like to see her continuing to write but I'd also like to see her continuing to be able to put photographs up."

Sarah: "David Payne thank you very much."

The interview had lasted three minutes. I ran upstairs to Rebecca.

"Was that OK?"

"It was great. Well done."

The previous night's planning had paid off and there were ticks on the crib sheets against the phrases I'd used. It was too soon to listen back on the BBC iPlayer but I was confident I'd got the important messages across. Scotland had its own morning news and current affairs radio programme and I accepted their interview request and at 8.19am I spoke to Good Morning Scotland. In the kitchen listening Joe was wondering if there was a delay as sound travelled along phone lines and airwaves. Polly was shouting, "It's Dad. It's Dad!" but Martha sat in silence.

I came back in and gave her a hug.

"It's done love. That's it. No more interviews." I sensed she was nervous being spoken about. "It was important to get the facts out. People are interested and I've made sure everyone knows the school is not to blame. Look at this," I added, taking her hand and sitting her in front of the computer. "Every cloud has a silver lining and in this case it's Mary's Meals. Look at the donations!"

She leant forward, turned and grinned.

"It's over £4500! We might make it!"

Even though Joe and Polly had heard every word from around the corner she rushed over and told them again.

The slide away from routine saw everyone in a mad dash of school bags, teeth and hair desperate to be ready on time for

school and work. There seemed no reason for Martha not to go to school along with her brother and sister and so, as it had since the start of the blog, life went on as usual.

Normality was soon to become in short supply. The neverseconds@gmail.com address I had given out on the Goodbye post was suddenly inaccessible from my phone. Emails were coming in at more than a 1000 an hour and even the computer was struggling. The page was scrolling so fast with new emails that I had to randomly click and wait to see which email opened. The emails weren't just offering support. People had taken action and were reporting the complaint they had made to Argyll and Bute council or the emails to politicians they had sent. I learnt later that the elected leader of the council, Roddy McCuish, had received calls from both the local member of the Scottish Parliament and the office of Alex Salmond, the First Minister of the Scottish Government by 8.30am. I was yet to find any support for the action of the council and the small amount of credibility they were clinging to was about to be shattered by their press release on the subject. Released onto their website was the following statement:

'Argyll and Bute Council wholly refutes the unwarranted attacks on its schools catering service which culminated in national press headlines which have led catering staff to fear for their jobs. The council has directly avoided any criticism of anyone involved in the 'never seconds' blog for obvious reasons despite a strongly held view that the information presented in it misrepresented the options and choices available to pupils however this escalation means we had to act to protect staff from the distress and harm it was causing. In particular, the photographic images uploaded appear to only represent a fraction of the choices available to pupils, so a decision has been made by the council to stop photos being taken in the school canteen.

There have been discussions between senior council staff and Martha's father however, despite an acknowledgement that the media coverage has produced these

unwarranted attacks, he intimated that he would continue with the blog.

The council has had no complaints for the last two years about the quality of school meals other than one from the Payne family received on 6 June and there have been no changes to the service on offer since the introduction of the blog.

Pupils have a daily choice of two meals from a menu which is designed with pupils, parents and teachers. Our summer menu is about to be launched and includes main course choices like meat or vegetarian lasagne served with carrots and garlic bread or chicken pie with puff pastry, mashed potato and mixed vegetables.

Pupils can choose from at least two meals every day. They pay £2 for two courses and this could be a starter and a main or a main and a desert. Each meal comes with milk or water. Pupils can have as much salad and bread as they want. Salad, vegetables, fruit, yoghurt and cheese options are available every day. These are standing options and are not a result of any changes in response to the blog site.

As part of the curriculum for excellence, pupils in all our schools are regularly taught about healthy eating and at lunch breaks staff encourage pupils to make good choices from what is on offer. We use a system called 'Nutmeg' to make sure everything is nutritionally balanced. Our staff also get nutrition awareness training so they know how to provide a good healthy meal. There is portion sized guidance which we adhere to and it is matched to the age of the child so they get the right amount of food. Second portions would mean too many calories for pupils.

In Lochgilphead Primary School we are piloting a new pre-ordering scheme which is designed to encourage class discussion around meal choices and also improves the accuracy of meal choices. The pupils use a touch screen

to select their lunch option and the data is downloaded in the kitchen so they know how many portions of each meal are required. As they place their order, the pupils are given a coloured band which relates to their meal choice that day. They wear it during the morning, and at lunchtime they hand it to the catering assistant, who will give them the corresponding meal.

The council's focus is now on supporting the school in the education of young people in Argyll and Bute'

It was couched in exactly the same terms that Cleland Sneddon had used on the phone. I immediately felt relief. Both my interviews that morning had been positive towards the school and whilst clearly in disagreement with the decision I had remained dignified. The press release was convoluted, angry and inaccurate. It was so bad it was wonderful. The text was immediately being dissected across twitter and respected blogger Adrian Short and Daily Telegraph journalist Tom Chivers took it apart word by word. There was no need for me to comment and so I sat watching Argyll and Bute continue to trend on twitter for all the wrong reasons whilst above it trended NeverSeconds and Mary's Meals for all the right ones.

The hospital, local newspaper office and swimming pool were deluged with calls trying to contact us. I was informed Scottish Television, BBC and Sky news were all sending camera crews. The story was a lead news item across all BBC radio stations and it looked like TV news wanted in on the action. At 10am Jamie Oliver, who had 2.5 million followers, tweeted.

'Stay strong Martha, RT this to show your support #neverseconds http://t.co/B1VlV7ak Jx'

He had encouraged all his followers to share the message by retweeting it and he had included a link to Martha's Goodbye post. NeverSeconds was getting more than 150,000 hits an hour as the Guardian also encouraged its readers to post their #mylunchformartha to show their support. With the internet leaping to Martha's defence I decided hiding was my best option

and leaving the constantly ringing home phone behind I fled to hide at Hazel and Steve's house in Ardrishaig a mile down the coast.

Hazel was following #neverseconds on twitter on her laptop calling out the names of supporters.

"That's Jay Rayner... Fleet Street Fox... Emma Kennedy... Rory Cellan-Jones... George Monbiot.... I can't keep up Dave!"

For every name I recognised there were thousands of ordinary people expressing their outrage. There was no doubt where public opinion lay and the comfort it brought was huge. I was knotted with stress. Unable to sit or stand comfortably I was pacing around the room. I was worried for Martha. My core belief that councils take their responsibilities seriously was shattered and I feared the Council would confront her again. Phone calls were becoming a welcome distraction.

"I'm sorry but I won't be doing an interview," I told the researcher at the Victoria Derbyshire show on BBC Radio 5 Live for the second time. I was starting to see the pushy side of the press. When the phone rang again I knew immediately that it was an attempt to trick me onto the programme. I could hear Victoria presenting the show not the researcher and so I cut off the call. Radio 5 is not easy to receive in the wilds of Argyll but Hazel managed to find it on the television and we listen to Cleland Sneddon give an interview. I was horrified. Time and time again he referred to the telephone call from the day before and he was happy to describe in detail what I had said. Considering I was part of that phone call I expected to recognise the conversation he was reporting. I did not. In response to a complaint I later made it was unfortunate his ability to recall the conversation with such clarity had deserted him and due to lack of evidence, it was his word against mine, the complaint was not upheld. My frustration however was short lived. At 12.18pm the JustGiving total went through £14,000.

Rebecca hadn't got my message that I was at Hazel's and arrived home for lunch only to find three cars parked neatly in front of the house. The BBC TV news team had found us. She dashed in and tried desperately to get me on my mobile but couldn't get through. It was half an hour before a text got to me

and I learned of the situation. By this time she had discussed our predicament with the BBC producer and it seemed the best approach might be for me to do an interview with them. It was a defensive measure. If I didn't give a television interview the various crews would continue to seek one and we might have ended up with more than three cars outside. It was a decision we had to take quickly.

"Dave, it's lifted! Roddy McCuish just did a u-turn!"

Hazel had kept half an ear on the lunchtime Radio 4 news World at One programme and live on air Roddy McCuish had reversed the decision. The presenter seemed shocked and took a moment to continue. It seemed that Roddy McCuish had wrestled the power away from council employees and used common sense to right a wrong. I knew I should have felt relief but I couldn't. The damage inflicted upon Martha and my family wasn't as easy to reverse as the decision on photography. Outside my house a TV crew waited whilst the decision makers whose actions had dragged Argyll and Bute Council's name through the mud hid in their offices away from prying eyes. A luxury their actions had removed from us.

The news networks reported the reversal as a breaking story and the combined national and international press now wanted to meet the girl who had defeated the council. We needed to get Martha, Joe and Polly home quickly and secretly. A plan was hatched and Hazel set off to collect the kids early to avoid an end of school day press scrum and I headed home to meet the BBC.

The BBC crew and presenter were smartly dressed, sharp and full of praise for Martha's blog. It was early afternoon and deadlines needed to be met. Crumpled haired from a sleepless night and in a day old shirt I allowed myself to be positioned for the camera and James Cook interviewed me. Some footage was filmed of us wandering and chatting to link scenes together and then as quickly as they had arrived they set off to Oban to meet Roddy McCuish. The item aired on the BBC1 6 o'clock news and on Reporting Scotland. Hazel had managed to smuggle the kids past the film crew at the school gates, though we later realised the crew weren't trying to film the kids, they were filming the school sign. Reuniting at Hazel's house was a chance to reflect

on the day.

"How was it kids?"

"It was ok," Martha said. "Bit strange at lunchtime though."

"It's been strange here too. The newspapers have been asking to speak to you and so have the television crews. Your story has been on the news all day and the council have changed their minds."

The news she could blog again brought a smile.

"Did we make it? Will there be a kitchen?"

"Oh yes, a kitchen and so much more."

I showed her the total.

It was 3.23pm and the JustGiving.com/NeverSeconds page had just whizzed past £28,000. It had doubled in 3 hours.

"Mary's Meals have asked for a photo though because you've raised so much money and they'd like to use it in a press release."

We slipped out onto the decking and using a camera phone I snapped Martha giggling as Hazel pulled faces behind my back. The photo went to Mary's Meals and then around the world.

Not only were we inundated but Nick Nairn was also. On a previous engagement in Glasgow he ended up at the BBC headquarters giving interviews in support of Martha's blog and against the decision to ban her. Having met Martha the day before he knew first hand there was no malice in her. Nick's day didn't end until after midnight with his last interview being given to a South American journalist whilst ours thankfully ended earlier. Not seeing the montage of Martha's photographs played to end Newsnight on BBC2 to the song 'Feed me' from the Little Shop of Horrors was my only regret. Martha's regret was simple.

"Shame I didn't take the camera. It was a good lunch today."

FRIDAY 15TH JUNE 2012

I think you know why I don't have a picture today but I will have on Monday! Thanks to everyone that has helped to get my blog back on track. I would have missed writing it a lot and I'm looking forward to sharing my dinners and yours.

I worried yesterday that I would never reach enough money to buy a Mary's Meal kitchen in Malawi (31 seconds!) but we have raised a total of £45,889.46 which is more than one kitchen! It could be many kitchens or one kitchen feeding many children for years.

A small thank you isn't enough so here's a big THANK YOU to you all!

See you on Monday,

VEG

Saturday 16th June

"Morning," I offered to the manager in the newsagent as I squeezed past to the news stand.

"You'll be wanting one of everything today. Hope you've got a big bag."

Looking at the rack I saw what he meant. Martha was front page on five of the Saturday newspapers and wasn't far behind in the rest. Picking a copy of each I was glad I'd come in early. Despite a good night I was still tired and my conversation with the manager was about as much as I could cope with.

"I've the same pile under the counter for the council to collect on Monday. That'll keep them busy."

"Aye it will."

I hurried home keen to avoid bumping into anyone. My confidence was waning under the strain of the coverage. The headlines recognised the worldwide support that had flowed into Lochgilphead. It was great that although Martha was the figurehead of the campaign it was in fact the pressure from Twitter, Facebook and the mainstream media that had saved the day.

NeverSeconds had sailed through 4 million hits and it was now receiving 44,000 hits an hour, twelve a second. The rising total on JustGiving was reflecting the care and concern that the world had for Martha and people were expressing it by donating to the cause that was closest to her heart. Every £10.70 that came in was going to provide a school meal for a year for a child somewhere that desperately needed it. Yes Martha could return to blogging but more importantly there were children who were going to be less hungry.

Martha was still sleeping upstairs as I began to tackle the

mountain of comments that needed moderation and emails that had come in. The coverage cycle was starting again but unlike last time we were contactable directly. NeverSeconds@gmail.com inbox was telling me I had 9,758 unread emails. I started answering each email and labelling them as I went for reference later. I marked emails as support, media, photo for blog or opportunity. I managed to get through 40 or so before Martha appeared at the door yawning.

"Are they for me?" she said, struggling to focus on the bright computer display.

"All of them are. There are nearly 10,000 emails for you to read." I pulled out some examples for her. She started to read out loud.

"Dear Veg. I am a producer with a television network in America and we would like to invite you to come and talk to us about your blog and visit the premiere of the new Disney movie 'Brave' about a Scottish girl. We think you are very brave. We know it is a long way to travel and so we are willing to provide flights and accommodation."

She looked at me wide eyed. "Can I go, Dad, can I?"

"I'm not sure it's a good idea love. I don't know the company. You know we tell you not to speak with strangers, well, this company are strangers to us. We don't know anything about them."

"You're so mean to me. I want to go."

"There will be fun things love but do you really want to travel for days just to see a film?"

Nine year olds don't picture the early flight check-ins, the waiting in airports or the scrum for a seat when they are imagining a film premiere in Hollywood. Just getting there would be a journey further than any we had undertaken before. The bigger issues to me were leaving behind the rest of the family. The invitation, as with most we were receiving, was for Martha and me. As relaxed as Joe and Polly were to wave their sister off on a holiday, it would only be divisive and no parent wishes to separate out one child as special or more important than another. The invitations within the UK certainly had less travel and more opportunity for the whole family to get involved.

"Last time you said you didn't like the idea of live TV."

"I was going to do Newsround, remember?"

Indeed it had been planned but Newsround had pulled out at the last minute. They were supposed to have been with us the day the council banned the photographs. I wondered if the producers were kicking themself now. It was from our experiences with Newsround that we were hesitant to get involved again. Martha had been excited and when the email came through cancelling it was of course my job to break it to her. The world had simply moved onto other topics in the eyes of Newsround but to Martha she had been let down. A promise had been broken and she felt it particularly hard when she had looked forward to it so much.

"I think people get excited and have great ideas but it's hard to make the ideas work sometimes. Look at this one."

I opened another email. This one suggested Martha should meet Michelle Obama, the first lady. Again it was from a news organisation in America.

"Who's she?" Martha asked.

"She's the American President Barack Obama's wife. She's tackling children's health and food issues in the States."

"Well if it's helping kids we should go."

"But the TV crew want us to do it so they can sell the film and get more people to watch their adverts. Someone's making money out of it. They are not doing it of the goodness of their hearts. It's the people being generous on your JustGiving page that are doing it selflessly."

Maybe it was because it was early and she was still bleary eyed or maybe it was because she was nine but either way a debate on altruism and the ethics of the press was not holding her attention. Turning she walked past the pile of newspapers without a glance and settled with a book in the conservatory.

Working through 1000's of emails was time consuming. I was replying personally to each and every one but emails were arriving quicker than I could reply. I wasn't even treading water. I was sinking. Searching the inbox for 'media' reduced the number of emails to just over three hundred but lost were the emails from grass root supporters. The answer to most of the requests was to be no. Sesame Street appearance? No thank you. Interview for Sunday Times? Ok. Offer to review fast food outlets for a

tabloid. No thanks. Interview on ABC Radio Australia? Not Martha, just me. I kept at it on and off during the day taking the practised approach of politeness and saying no quickly so papers and TV could move on to another plan.

By evening I had replied to all the emails; spoken to the majority of the Sunday papers and provided the photograph of Martha on Hazel's decking to all requests. Glancing at Twitter I could see there was great excitement about a video on YouTube and following the link I was soon staring at a tartan covered wall with a large map of Scotland pinned to it. I was watching Argyll & Bute - The NeverSeconds Song by the Scottish Falsetto Sock Puppet Theatre by Kev Sutherland. To the tune of Mull of Kintyre by Paul McCartney the puppets started singing.

'Argyll & Bute
Forbid a wee girl photographing her food
And ban her from blogging from
Argyll & Bute
Dull was the pizza and few were the peas
So Martha aged nine took some photos of these
Up on her blog her school dinners she put
And was banned by the council of
Argyll & Bute'

The pile of papers lay forgotten as I was joined first by Rebecca and then by the kids laughing our way through our own recital of the NeverSeconds Song.

MONDAY 18TH JUNE 2012

Friends of NeverSeconds

Kitchen here we come! We have raised £85,429.63 so far but I am unsure if I should add the Gift Aid at the bottom of the JustGiving page. That means a whole kitchen in Lirangwe Primary School in Blantyre, Malawi (8 seconds I'm getting good at Malawi!) and enough left over to feed another 5800 dinners to other children! Mary's Meals asked me what I would like to call the kitchen and I said 'Friends of NeverSeconds' because if it was just me I would never have managed to raise enough but now we have!

I always choose the lamb meatballs when they are on the menu. Everyone gets the same number of balls because it's fair. Today we had 5. The gravy is hard to eat with a knife and fork but it is nice with the meatballs and the mash potato. There is one piece of cucumber missing because I ate it before the photograph! The dessert is called Golden Crunchie and I think it has syrup and cornflakes in it. It's one of the sticky puddings so I use a spoon so I don't have to waste any lunch break washing my hands.

Food-o-meter- 8/10
Mouthfuls- forty something
Courses- main/dessert
Health Rating- 8/10 because I don't know what's in the meatballs
Price- £2
Pieces of hair- 0
Ease of eating with wrist in stookie- 10/10
Wristband- Orange

Alexandra is 18 and goes to school at SHAPE High School in Belgium (21 seconds, it's shortened to Belg on my globe). She says 'This is a NATO base and we have many international students here! We all go to school together. They are really pushing the healthy aspect, so we do not get as much as we used to do (portion-wise). We had 3 choices today. I chose the chicken patty.'

Food-o-meter: 8/10
Mouthfuls: 42 (I didn't really eat it all)
Courses: main/dessert
Heath Rating: 8/10
Price: 2 Euros
Pieces of Hair: 0

I think a patty is a burger, the tube by the banana is a yoghurt and I do not know what is in the Ranch packet!

VEG

Monday 18th June

Ignoring phones and emails for Father's Day had seemed like a very good idea at the time and along with friends from the Triathlon club we had spent an enjoyable day swimming in the old slate quarries on Easdale Island up the coast from Lochgilphead. The clear waters separated from the Atlantic by a thin wall of remaining island rock are atmospheric, with reminders of the island's industrial past surrounding you. But it seemed rude to walk away from the rising total on JustGiving. Martha and I had started to reply individually to every donation she received but the task soon became unmanageable. For once Martha was being allowed to not write her thank you letters and in the circumstances I felt people would understand. Each donation was accompanied by a comment and Martha and I spent time reading them to each other.

"What's the Streisand effect Dad?"

A donor had commented on seeing the Streisand effect in action.

"Best Google it," I suggested.

Together we read the Wikipedia entry on how Barbara Streisand had taken legal action to force the removal of a photograph from a website of her home. The photograph had been viewed six times before the legal action. The publicity resulted in 420,000 visits to website in the following month.

"Dad, Dad! Look!" Martha was pointing to the list of examples and there at the bottom was NeverSeconds with a link to a BBC article.

"Your blog's got a mention on Wikipedia. Wow."

Martha was already typing NeverSeconds into the search box and up appeared a comprehensive entry on the blog.

"Ha, I'm going to show my friends at school. They can't see the blog but they can see this."

It was a shame that NeverSeconds was banned at her school. We were receiving lots of emails from schools where her blog was part of class daily routine. Some were using it as part of world food topics, others in English as a foreign language lessons. We even found a page where ten words had been removed from her post and the aim was to fill them in as an online homework task for a Spanish school. Disappointingly I only got eight out of ten and Martha trumped me with a nine. The continued council blocking of her blog ran counter to their assertion that they did not want to censor Martha and left Martha surrounded by rumour in the playground instead of fact. The Streisand effect had certainly played its part though and a look at the photograph statistics showed 34,488,899 images had been viewed. I wondered what the total would have been if the blog was visible across Argyll and Bute Council controlled networks.

The Scotland on Sunday broadsheet newspaper had carried the headline: 'We love Martha. How a 9-year-old from Argyll won the nation's heart', with a full page analysis inside from Dani Garavelli. We were through the first part of the coverage cycle of raw news reported fast and getting into a more analytical stage. Commentators were keen to point out the council's actions were a lesson in how not to behave and I was repeatedly being asked to discuss my interactions with the council and school. The international ridicule that Argyll and Bute Council had brought upon itself, the stress and damage they had caused to Martha and our family along with the 3894 complaints it had received was, I hoped, a catalyst for change. I expected that the start of a new week would bring news of a resignation or an enquiry. It was for the council to put its own house in order and I refused to be drawn into fuelling the mass condemnation of their actions.

Martha headed to school not full of news of front-page photographs, which for the third day in the row was the case, but with excitement that Mary's Meals were going to be able to build a kitchen in Malawi. The honour of naming the kitchen was hers and with the story continuing to dominate, Mary's Meals were keen to announce the name and capitalise on the interest.

"Think about it and tell me when you get home! Remember we've visitors from Mary's Meals after school."

"Martha's kitchen!"

I started to protest.

"Joking," she called, slamming the car door, and I hoped she was.

Mary's Meals had generously offered us its support and as the phone started its incessant call I was very grateful for it. Common sense had got us this far safely but the pressures to hear from Martha on television were mounting. The unwillingness to put Martha out there made her an even bigger prize, which was being pursued tirelessly from all corners. I received a call from the Jeremy Vine show on BBC Radio, a lunchtime show mixing music with interviews and phone ins.

"No I won't discuss the council or their decision. Happy to talk about the positives and the incredible fund raising total for Mary's Meals. That's it," I told the researcher.

She was pleased with that and we spent the next fifteen minutes discussing the cost of supporting a child for a year and the ins and outs of building a kitchen in Malawi. I was looking forward to sharing the charity and its good work and was waiting to go live when the producer said:

"Thanks for waiting, Mr Payne. You're on next and Roddy McCuish will follow you."

With a sinking feeling I realised I had been played. Knowing I wouldn't talk about the council they had tricked me into appearing by giving the impression it was to be about Mary's Meals. Jeremy's questions were so fast there was no time to mention the charity and all I could do was concentrate on being supportive to the school and the dinner ladies. Thankfully my crumpled crib sheet was still in my pocket and I was able to be as uncontroversial as I could. I did not mention the offensive phone call nor the terrible press release. As a family we had survived so far on our wits but feeling deceived by a well-known BBC programme was sign enough that we needed good advice quickly. Mary's Meals has an experienced staff including an ex BBC Scotland journalist who were not surprised at the tactics taken and we gladly accepted their offer of support.

I could now forward all emails and direct phone calls to

Mary's Meals Dalmally headquarters. The connection between NeverSeconds and Mary's Meals was understood by the press and for the first time we were able to lighten the load. It was no longer just down to me to say no, and requests from The Lorraine Show and others were handled sensitively on our behalf. Already we were being asked if we would be travelling to Malawi and I had been clear that we weren't planning a trip. A summer of camping was planned and an autumn trip to the south of France already booked.

Meeting the staff from Mary's Meals made a huge impression on Martha. She heard first hand stories about how the money would change lives for children. Children her age were working for survival and missing out on education. A simple meal was in many cases a life saver. Completing the gaps in her knowledge made Martha more determined to share the work of Mary's Meals on her blog. It was athletics club time and we had to make our farewells and thank yous too soon. As Martha ran, jumped and threw at the club I was receiving emails questioning where that day's post was. The world was waiting and getting impatient. Once home she started. I was distracted as she typed and when she passed it over for me to read I saw she'd decided to call the kitchen 'Friends of NeverSeconds'.

"Are you alright, Dad?"

All the pride and love I felt for her welled up in my eyes and unable to hide it I just gave in and allowed big tears to roll down my face.

"Friends of NeverSeconds. That's perfect."

Martha twisted on her seat, hugged me and added, "Thought so."

TUESDAY 19TH JUNE 2012

Mini Olimpicz

If you think I have spelt Olympics wrong I haven't! The word Olympics is copyrighted so the school would get a fine if we used it. There were lots of sports but some I missed because of my stookie but it was fun rolling on the paddling pool to get the air out.

I wanted to try a tuna baked potato because I have never had one at school before but I have had them at home. I didn't eat the skin of the potato because it was soft and I like them crisp. The carrots and salad were nice and crunchy and the tuna was soft. The soup is always hot so I tend to eat it at the end. The mugs we have for soup are blue like the Mary's Meals mugs which the children use but ours are smaller. The soup was chicken noodle but I don't think it has actual chicken but it doesn't matter because it's lovely without.

Martha Payne and David Payne

Food-o-meter- 9/10
Mouthfuls- 46
Courses- starter/main
Health Rating- 9/10
Price- £2
Pieces of hair- 0
Ease of eating with wrist in stookie- 8/10 it was hard to get the potato out of its skin
Wristband- Purple

I am thrilled that the total on our JustGiving page for Mary's Meals is £91,409.00. It means so much. It's almost 10,000 children receiving a school dinner for a year! Dad sang a song in the car about someone called Lola because a donation came from Barry Manilow. I recognised the song!

VEG

Tuesday 19th June

'Had I heard of Noma?' an email from Copenhagen asked me. A watcher of MasterChef, I had seen the episode where the finalists had cooked in Noma, currently the best restaurant in the world for the third year running. The food was imaginative and sourced from a range of fantastic foraged ingredients. I read on hopeful and was not disappointed. Martha and I were being invited, all expenses, to stay in Copenhagen for the weekend of their annual MAD (Danish for food) conference for chefs. The list of attendees was a who's who of the best chefs in the world and included Hugh Fearnley-Whittingstall whose River Cottage series of books had inspired me to try smallholding. We were being invited to give a ten-minute talk on appetite, the theme of the conference. Using Skype I chatted with Chef René Redzepi who was excited that Martha had such a passion for food and wanted her to share and inspire the chefs. It was a wonderful and kind opportunity and one I wanted to take up. The weekend of the conference was the first weekend of the school holidays and we were all free. Bringing the rest of the family would be no bother and what a way for Martha to enjoy some success from her hard work.

For the first time in days I had a spring in my step. The support from Mary's Meals meant I could answer emails of support and leave the media related ones to them. We'd managed a long discussion with Mary's Meals about what we were comfortable with. Important to us was not to try and turn the situation we were in into a money-making opportunity. From a young age our children had learnt that we give them what they need rather than what they want. Christmas in our house was a much quieter affair than many, with only small presents. We always

visited the hospital on Christmas Day, when I became Santa and the children elves to put a smile on the patients' faces and drop off Chocolate Oranges for the staff. Many of the patients were elderly and they particularly like to see children at Christmas. So to try and make as much money out of the flurry of interest went against the grain and such offers were easy to decline.

There were opportunities that we were happy to support, though. When The Children's Food Trust, a charity, got in touch I readily agreed to speak at their conference the following year. Likewise a food photography competition that asked Martha to be their young ambassador got our support. Martha's interest in what she ate had grown since she started photographing her food and we wanted to encourage other children to have the same experience. There were fun things ahead and it was looking brighter.

Whilst I was smiling at home things were taking a turn for the worse at school. Playtime and lunch were becoming a chance for Martha to be the focus of bullying and a number of unkind and generally older boys were making it hard for her to continue to enjoy school in the way she normally did. The act of banning the blog had sowed the seed in young minds that Martha needed to be punished. Martha had been treated with respect, kindness and fairness by teacher and dinner lady alike and this was witnessed by every child in the school and the good example of the staff had been followed until now. But when the council made its attacks on Martha and her blog it undermined the work of the school staff and the tone in school changed. Every time Martha had to stand up to the bullies alone her confidence took a tiny knock. As the incidences increased the little knocks became larger dents. The smile so ready to spring across her face took a second longer to appear. Whilst Roddy McCuish attempted to fix the reputation of the council with promises of summer school dinner summits with Nick Nairn, no attempt was being made by the council to repair the damage to Martha's reputation they had caused. Martha had never received an apology either in person or by email or letter. No leader of the council stood up in her school praising her fund raising achievement to help restore her good name in front of her peers. She was instead abandoned to fend for herself

within a hostile atmosphere generated through the incompetent actions of the council.

The pressure I had been bearing from the media was now being experienced by the Mary's Meals staff. If anything, interest was intensifying and there were a growing number of feature requests for a longer interview with Martha and the family. There was always the worry that if we did not cooperate then some papers would still run a piece based on whatever they could glean locally about us. At least if we spoke to a paper on our terms we had some control over what was written. Mary's Meals suggested that we worked with a journalist from the Daily Telegraph. The paper was a long-time supporter of the charity and with their contacts within the paper they could guarantee that the article, whilst needing to recognise the origins of the story, would give equal weight to the positive outcome for Mary's Meals. The Telegraph was also willing to send a film crew along. The video footage would be on the Telegraph website, made available to Mary's Meals free of charge and also released to the world's media. It seemed the only way to pull the safety valve on the simmering situation and we agreed to the arrangement.

I was determined that although I was nervous about the visit from the Telegraph I was not going to show it to the girls. In the car on the way home I shared the fun news of the day.

"I've been chatting to Noma. Best restaurant in the world," I told Martha and Polly who both looked at me blankly.

"The one from the MasterChef final," I added.

Clearly Noma had made a far greater impression on me than them. I explained the chance we had to go and visit.

"But that's the first weekend of our holiday. We're camping with Grannie Annie and Grandpa Barry," Martha recalled.

"They won't mind. They'll understand."

"Will you be terribly upset," Martha started, "if we don't go. I'd rather go camping."

It had taken Martha's honesty to remind me that in a nine-year-old girl's life camping with Grannie and Grandpa was far more exciting than the world's best restaurant, and when I told René at Noma about her words we laughed together.

WEDNESDAY 20TH JUNE 2012

I met two ladies from Mary's Meals who told me children
have to walk for 2 hours to get to their school every day.
I couldn't walk that far every day. The kitchens start
cooking early in the morning so that all the children get
fed so thanks again for your support!

Today's meal was delicious. It was a beef burger, roast
potatoes and peas. I didn't want any salad today. The
roast potatoes were soft. The ice lolly for dessert
comes in orange, yellow, purple and green. I got given
purple. It has two sticks because it's easier to hold that
way.

Food-o-meter- 10/10
Mouthfuls- 32 not including licks.
Courses- main/dessert
Health Rating- 2/10
Price- £2
Pieces of hair- 0
Ease of eating with wrist in stookie- 5/10 hard to hold
ice lolly
Wristband- Orange

I got this fantastic email from Australia,

We are from a school in Australia (in Nowra – on the
south coast of New South Wales, 21 seconds!). We found
out about your blog from one of our teachers who is
from Scotland, like you! How cool is that??!! At school in
Australia most kids have to bring their lunch from home.
Some schools have a canteen where students can buy
their lunch, but our school is too small to have a canteen.
So we do cooking every second Wednesday instead.

Today was cooking day and we cooked Salmon Fish Cakes with Garlic Mayonnaise and Lemon. It was DELICIOUS!

Here are our scores (We have averaged our scores for the whole school, the serving was 2 fish cakes each):

Food-O-Meter: 9/10
Mouthfuls: 7
Courses: Main
Healthy Rating: 8.5/10
Price: AU$1.25 (BUT we used lemons from Mrs M's lemon tree and an egg from the school chickens)
Pieces of Hair: 0 (thank goodness!)

We think your blog is great, and we love how you raise money for kids in Africa. We pay for our cooked lunch ($2 each) and we are using it to raise money for a clean water well in Cambodia (through Samaritan's Purse).

From,
Steven and Nicholas (Primary 2 — year 1 in Australia!)

Andrew (Primary 5 — year 4)

Mrs G

Mrs M (who's from Scotland!)'

I would really enjoy eating your homemade fishcakes. It's great you get to cook. We sometimes do too. It's so cool you have school chickens!

VEG

Wednesday 20th June

I wondered what first impressions a Daily Telegraph writer and cameraman would have arriving in Argyll. The remoteness had worked in our favour when news editors were making decisions on whether to send a camera crew on the off chance they would be able to get footage. Had we lived in Glasgow or Edinburgh our doorstep would have been more heavily trod than it was. Most commented on by visitors was the space we all enjoy. Surrounded by heather clad hill, lochs and forests, a network of trails gave us miles of exploring. With a cloudless sky the sun brought Loch Fyne to life and as the road swept past the sea to Lochgilphead the jagged outline of Arran was visible in the distance. After the tightness of London the breadth of Argyll was relaxing in itself and our journalist visitors were to arrive smiling despite the long journey.

Nerves were making smiles rarer at home. Sharing our home with friends was easy but sharing it with journalists was not. Our quirky house spread over three floors reflected our characters. Practicality ruled over looks and cycling helmets lay alongside running shoes in the hall. The kitchen had colour swatches on the wall from a burst of decorating enthusiasm from over a year ago. How the chaotic homeliness would be reported we did not know and a morning of cleaning and sorting had done little to lighten the mood. Thankfully Granny Jane and Grandpa John were on their way. The kids were very lucky to have two sets of grandparents so different in their outlooks and ways. The excitement of camping with my parents was balanced with Jane and John's ability to make every day special with arts and crafts. We needed their calmness today. I had been tetchy that morning getting the kids out the door for school and though

normally it's guaranteed the kids come home from school happy the attention Martha was getting now was changing things.

Leaving Rebecca at home to make the introductions I collected the kids from school. Little detective work from me was needed to work out that the downturn at school had continued. Slumped shoulders replaced Martha's normal strong stride. The car was not the place to practice my soft skills so instead I sang.

"Her name was Lola…"

"Dad, you did this yesterday," Martha grumped back.

"So join in. Her name was Lola, she was a show girl… oh come on its Barry Manilow! He donated to your page yesterday. Least we can do is sing."

Polly joined in and the two of us stumbled through repeated choruses until we were home. Failing to raise Martha's mood did not bode well for the impending interview and filming.

Miraculously where I had failed, Granny Jane did not. On seeing Granny Martha leapt from the car, dashed down the steps to the patio and leapt onto Granny's knee, smiling.

It was clear that Martha wasn't completely relaxed with strangers amongst us and being wired for a radio microphone isn't the icebreaker you might think it is. Soon though, with chat about pets and friends the atmosphere lightened and the Telegraph writer did get to see the side of Martha that we all know. Martha described the school in Lirangwe outside Blantyre where the 'Friends of NeverSeconds' kitchen was to be built and the different lives the children who attended it had to lead.

"Will you visit the school?" asked the Telegraph.

"I'd like to but…"

"Sorry Martha. Won't happen."

I'd cut her off rudely and harshly and everyone knew it but I'd seen the glance that had flicked between Grandpa John and Rebecca. Martha was not for taking a hint.

"It would be fun. I'd like to meet all the children and say hi."

The pupils had sent a video message to Martha and she'd shared it on the blog. They were smiling, excited and inviting. Martha wasn't expressing a desire to be thanked. She was seeing a happy picture that she wanted to be part of.

The journalistic experience that Martha wanted when asking to write everyday was becoming very real. Her daily blogging

was now coming on top of interviews and phone calls. As the end of any school term approached the kids became more tired and with the extra end of year evening activities it was becoming hard for Martha to find the time to write. Her enthusiasm for her own school dinner was being eroded because lunchtime was when she was hardest pushed by the bullies. It was no longer a pleasant break in the day to enjoy some food; it was now a time she was beginning to dread. Her photographs had always come home as one shot but now there were many out of focus because she was being jostled as she tried to take it. With every blurred failure she had to remain standing longer, compose the photo and take it again. To do it four times as she did one day showed strength and it was clear at home that the she was drawing some of that strength from the children in Malawi she was helping. Whenever she picked up the computer to blog she started by looking at the JustGiving page. It wasn't just the rising total that made her happy, it was the wonderfully kind comments. She showed me an example from Canada:

'It is Father's Day today. My kids asked me if it was ok to not go out to dinner to celebrate but to donate the cost instead to Mary's Meals. You are an inspiration Veg. Keep it up.'

The donation accompanying the comment was enough to feed five children for a year.

But coping with the mixed messages she was receiving was confusing her. Her blog readers were clear on the positive impact she was having on the school dinner debate nationally and internationally. Her JustGiving supporters were impressed that inspiration could come from someone so young. But the reaction coming from the council seemed dominated by their embarrassment and was mute because of it. Rating her dinner of beef burger, roast potatoes and peas 10/10 on the food-o-meter whilst it only got a 2/10 on its health rating was Martha's desperate attempt to appease her bullies. But the summer holidays were approaching and Martha's interest in her own school dinners was becoming surpassed by her interest in the school dinners sent in from around the world.

THURSDAY 21ST JUNE 2012

Concert

I had my stookie off today and tonight I have been in a concert so I have not had time to blog. Sorry! I hope we can celebrate raising £100,000 soon for Mary's Meals. We are so close. I don't know what I'll do!

VEG

Thursday 21st June

The interview and filming with the Daily Telegraph had taken it out of us all. The end of term could not come quick enough. Still a week to go and energy levels were starting to hit bottom. Waking the kids up for the start of each day was becoming harder and the morning routine seemed to be played out in slow motion. Martha's difficulties at school and Rebecca's increasingly stressful job were sucking away at the mirth we were used to having. Even Polly's comical antics weren't enough raise the collective mood.

Thankfully preventing us from sliding further was the incredible capacity people have to give. Even in hard times the willingness to share was reflected in the JustGiving donations. The thousands of contributions the friends of NeverSeconds were making was news around the world. More interview requests were becoming about Mary's Meals and the work they would be doing with the growing total. I had the key figures in my head that 650,000 children are fed daily in 16 countries and that £10.70 feeds a child for a year. Describing sponsoring a kitchen at a cost of £7000 took me to the limit of my knowledge and it was to Grandpa John that I turned for a better understanding.

Mary's Meals worked in collaboration with local communities in Malawi. It started with an invite to help the community feed its children and a partnership had developed. Land was usually donated for a kitchen shelter to be built on and when a sponsor was found local builders constructed it. Volunteers in Malawi organised the cooking rotas and in the early morning women carrying wood for the fires arrived to begin preparations. In Malawi it was likuni phala, a type of porridge made

from locally grown maize, soya and sugar supplemented with minerals and vitamins. Most of the children that queued outside the shelter would not have eaten before school and for many it was their only substantial meal of the day. Enrolment to the school increased when the partnership of local people and Mary's Meals began its work and the number of children passing their exams had increased.

Behind the simple solution to world hunger that Martha could understand lay a collaborative system supporting local communities to improve the future outlook for their children. The parallels between Martha's NeverSeconds and the work of Mary's Meals was uncanny and I could only be more impressed with the work of Mary's Meals the more I heard. I hoped to be able to follow the successful collaborative examples from Malawi with our own meeting with the council leader, which had been arranged before the photography ban fiasco.

As we drove through the arch and to the car park at the rear of the council headquarters I was still fielding phone calls from the press.

"I will not be doing a live interview after the meeting with you or any other news organisation," I told Sky News firmly. I had no idea how the meeting would pan out and I had no intention of appearing on camera.

John was nodding his agreement. Mary's Meals had advised us that it was likely that an attempt would be made to get me to comment. I had planned in my mind the polite lines I would use whilst walking past the cameras back to my car. Roddy McCuish along with his colleagues, local councillors Dougie Philand and Sandy Taylor, were waiting when we arrived and after handshakes all round we sat down to business. It was another unminuted meeting. Speaking frankly I described the telephone call Cleland Sneddon had given me. I received no reaction of surprise from the councillors. I outlined how, over a month ago, I had sat in the same building with Dougie Philand, Malcolm MacFadyen and Jayne Murphy, discussing our differences and agreeing to a joint press release. The council's missed opportunities when listed alongside their actions were embarrassing and so it was gratifying that the failings I had recounted were also recognised by the councillors.

The disastrous banning of Martha's photography and subsequent press release would not have happened, I was assured, if the councillors had been made aware of the plans. It left the question of who really was in charge of the council, the faceless bureaucrats or the elected members whose photos appeared in the local newspaper. Both John and I left the meeting with a strong sense that the need for change was recognised and that the difficult first steps along that road were already being taken. If the councillors could bring about the institutional attitude changes they sought it would be another good thing to have come from NeverSeconds.

Driving past the Joint Campus School the next day we were unaware that the bullying had reached new heights. As Martha attempted to have her lunch she was prevented from taking a photograph. The failure to remove the stigma of the ban had led to unchecked ugly scenes again. Phone calls were made to the school and assurances received. The head had been away and was unaware of the latest incident and things were to improve. When no photo appeared on her blog readers guessed correctly the cause even though Martha had decided herself not to write about the bullying. The reaction from her supporters would have been immediate and though the bullying was taking place in school the blame rested in the council offices. The upset Martha was feeling was soothed by a phone call from the BBC Radio Scotland newsroom.

"She's done it! She's only gone and done it! You are through the £100k well done! Got to go. On air. Bye!"

I missed the name of the caller whose excitement matched Martha's as she looked at the page. Sash Window Repair Man from Brighton had made a donation of £3000 with the comment:

'Martha, again well-done on everything. It was an absolute pleasure to donate to your cause, and utterly demolish that 100.000 barrier. I hope the news companies carry your 100k success and more donations continue to pour in over the weekend. Enjoy the party you deserve it.'

Martha danced around the house and the phone rang as the good news spread. It was a moment to celebrate, but how? Martha wanted to invite all her friends from Charity Children for a party but a table laden with food seemed at odds with the lives of the hungry children Martha was helping. Instead, Mary's Meals sent us some of the likuni phala and we celebrated as a family with steaming mugs of the porridge. The end of term was only days away and of course with no school dinners for Martha NeverSeconds would go silent.

"I'll miss seeing the school dinners from other countries," Martha said between slurps.

"Has it been fun, Martha? Would you recommend it?"

"It was fun until he banned it. I learnt lots."

"Maybe we should see if other children would like to share their dinners whilst you are on holiday."

I placed a request onto the blog and immediately was inundated with offers from children and schools to guest blog for a week at a time during the holidays. The enthusiasm was electric and Martha was excited to see the list of places the blog would be visiting.

FRIDAY 22ND JUNE 2012

It was too hard to take my photo today. I am going to
describe my meal instead. We always have the same trays.
On it today I had fish, chips and peas with a yoghurt and
some water. The fish was golden brown and very crunchy.
It was the the size of my hand but thinner. The fish
inside was white with bits of brown and grey. We don't
get vinegar or salt only tomato sauce which is served to
you on a spoon. I ate my chips with my fingers and dipped
them in the ketchup. The peas are hard to get on your
fork so I stabbed them.

Food-o-meter- 6/10
Mouthfuls- forgot to count
Courses- main/dessert
Health Rating- 5/10
Price- £2
Pieces of hair- 0
Wristband- Orange

We are going to Erlgasse school in Vienna, Austria (10
seconds!). English group 2bd, Marcus, Filip, Ana, Nici, Salih,
Alisha, Vivi, Musti, Sandra, Christopher, Sara, Laura, Meli,
Michelle, Can, Anita, Mehtap and their teacher Miss Killian
wrote,

'Our school is from eight o'clock till one or two clock most
days. Sometimes we have afternoon classes. Some pupils
go to after-school care and only these eat at school.
There is either salad or soup, and always a dessert.
Dessert is sometimes fruit, but we always get fruit one
hour after lunch.

This is Tuesday's lunch "Wurstsalat"

It's sausage meat mixed with tomato, cheese, lettuce, gherkins. Dessert was a raspberry pudding, but we don't have a picture of it.

Food-o-meter: 6 of 10
Mouthfuls- 34
Pieces of hair: 0
Health rating: 8 of 10
Price: EUR 4,20 (that's 3,39 in British Pounds)
Food tester: Kevin'

Your bread looks really dark and I like your Wurstsalat but it's really expensive!

I am planning a Porridge Party if we manage to raise over £100,000 for Mary's Meals. We are really close now so I hope we make it over the weekend!

VEG

VEG's Dad here.

School holidays start soon here in Scotland. We are looking for schools from around the world to guest blog on NeverSeconds and show us their daily dose of school dinners. For one week it's your chance to show us what's important to you about your lunch. If your class would like to take on the challenge please get in touch with NeverSeconds@gmail.com . Many thanks!

Martha Payne and David Payne

The Summer Holidays

All the guest bloggers followed Martha's example of choosing a pseudonym, photographing their school dinner and describing and rating their food.

Blodwyn from Anglesey, Wales, wrote beautifully in Welsh and was able to show readers a more positive UK school dinner experience. Blodwyn's school cook has gone on to win an award for her skills. Pride shone through all the guest bloggers' posts and robust debates raged in the comments section of the blog as to the relative health ratings given to the dinners. By sharing different international daily experiences kids were opening each other's eyes and were seeing how food is more important in some cultures than others. Particularly in Scotland and America the cult of convenience seemed to set the agenda. School dinners had to be convenient to prepare, to eat quickly and to clear up. The embarrassment that Martha's dinners had brought on Argyll and Bute Council reflected the low importance that Scottish and UK governments give to our children's school dinner experience.

Doni from Japan, guest blogging in September, highlighted the void in approaches between our two countries. We expected our school teachers to be great role models and to set an example for the pupils in their classrooms. By bowing to convenience and cost the example set in school dining halls had to be held responsible in part for the growing health issues our country faced. Martha's efforts were recognised again by Jamie Oliver who awarded NeverSeconds Blog of the Month on his Food Revolution website. NeverSeconds was being talked about in the corridors of power in Parliament in London and a motion in the Scottish Government read:

'Martha Payne's Blog Goes on Tour and Continues to Raise Money

That the Parliament recognises the contribution of the nine-year-old Lochgilphead pupil, Martha Payne, for her superb result in raising more than £110,000 through her blog, Never Seconds; understands that the blog is a daily comment on her school meals, through which she has managed to bring the attention of school pupils, staff and parents to matters of nutrition and school meals in a way that it considers famous chefs have failed to do; notes that the blog has attracted interest worldwide, has focused attention on issues across the globe and has also raised what it considers an amazing sum of money, which is still growing, to enable Mary's Meals, an Argyll-based charity, to provide for children in Malawi, and wishes Martha a happy and carefree summer holiday while her blog is taken over by other children around the world.'

With such glowing praise being heaped upon the blog it was easy to smile at the email from Argyll and Bute Council rejecting all of our complaints. I wondered if an independent investigation would draw the same conclusions but we had carried out our duty in pointing out where we felt their failures were and we could do no more.

The summer of 2012 will be remembered by many for the rain and our camping trips certainly tested the quality of our canvas. Camping had that element of adventure that the children loved and the drumming of rain on the tent wasn't stopping the kids from getting out to play on the campsite. We listened to the half hour BBC Radio Food programme that Martha had made earlier in the week with Sheila Dillon. Called the 'Extraordinary Food World of Martha Payne', our life on the smallholding was contrasted with the food served in schools. Martha and Polly were keener to meet our new neighbours than listen to themselves and watched in fascination as a family from Germany arrived on two motorbikes. Approaching as close as they dared our girls stood staring, as an invite, until the two children came over and

within minutes frisbee and tig games had started.

"They don't stop talking to each other even though they don't speak the same language do they," Rebecca pointed out to me.

The glance cast between Grandpa John and Rebecca hadn't been forgotten and the assumption in the press that we would visit the school in Lirangwe had been allowed to go unchecked. I waited for it.

"It'd be the same in Malawi."

"We've booked £1200 worth of flights to France. It's too much to lose," I answered back.

Mary's Meals had been very kind and contacted Ryanair on our behalf to see if a refund was possible considering the charitable aspect but the request was declined.

"Do you think we'll ever have an opportunity like this again? Martha seeing how her hard work has changed lives and you're not sure? Really?"

The root of Martha's determination was clear to see and an argument about cost seemed churlish against the priceless experience on offer.

"Grandpa wants to come to experience for himself how Mary's Meals works in Malawi. He hasn't done it yet because he didn't want to be a tourist getting in the way. There's a real purpose to this trip though."

Mary's Meals were encouraging and told us the press were interested in accompanying us. It wouldn't be selfish to visit if we could share the experience. Finally I realised that going was the right thing to do for Martha, the family and for Mary's Meals.

THURSDAY 28TH JUNE 2012

Porridge Party!

We have raised over £108,000 for Mary's Meals and to celebrate I had a Porridge Party! I cooked some Likuni Phala. I measured out the mixture and added the water. I kept stirring it as it cooked and it didn't stick. Mary's Meals told me,

'Porridge provides a delicious breakfast for people all over the UK, but for over 549,000 schoolchildren in Malawi it is a powerful incentive to go to school and, for many, the only nutritious meal they will have that day.

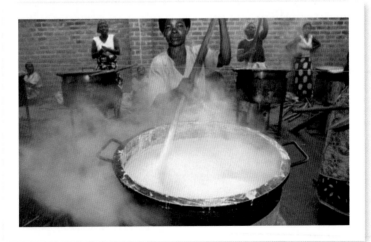

At schools in Malawi where Mary's Meals is working, every child is given a daily serving of likuni phala — which is a nutritious, vitamin—enriched maize porridge served in plastic mugs.

The porridge meets the children's immediate needs by filling their empty bellies, but also attracts them to the classroom where they can get an education which can lift them out of poverty in later life.

Each child is responsible for looking after their own mug, and holding on to it ensures they get a fair portion every school day. Some carry them around their necks on a piece of string to make sure they don't miss out.'

I really enjoyed the porridge. It's different to Scottish porridge and it's sweet and filling. Here I am tasting it! Remember it only costs 6p a day to feed a child with Mary's Meals. 6p.

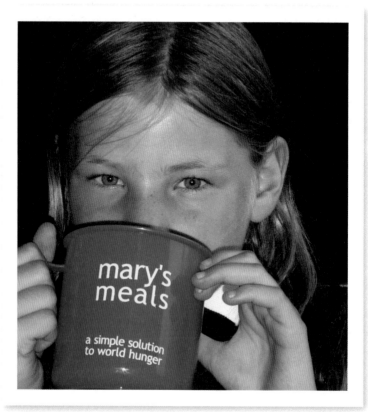

I can't believe I am going to Malawi later in the year to help finish the 'Friends of NeverSeconds' kitchen sign and meet the children receiving Mary's Meals. I want to blog everyday when I am there but dad isn't sure how we'll manage it! Meanwhile NeverSeconds will be on its travels. More on that tomorrow.

So here's me and my dad saying thanks to you all!

I want the last word to go to Jailosi who is 10 years old and from Blantyre in Malawi. He says,

"Likuni phala gives us energy to learn and walk back home after school. We also have the heart to come back to school the next day because we know we will have porridge. I tell everyone how Mary's Meals helps the weak to become strong."

VEG

SUNDAY 23 SEPTEMBER 2012

I'm so excited!

I have been talking to lots of people about going to Malawi. I'm talking a lot about it because I am excited about it. I have been told food on planes isn't very good but I hope they are wrong. I have never eaten a meal on a plane before. I don't think a plane has a kitchen it must be made on the ground and reheated in the air. I will rate my meals on the plane!

It's amazing how the kitchen has improved from a little shelter with a thatched roof to a building with walls and a metal roof. The next picture you see of the Friends of NeverSeconds kitchen will have me in it. I will be there! I will tell them how it happened that a blog built a kitchen.

I can't wait to meet all the children. I have packed some footballs and wind up torches. We don't have any Kwatcha for Malawi yet so we've no money. Dad says it's ok. Soon I start taking antimalarial tablets. I have to have 4 a day but my sister only has to have 1. It is because I am not quite an adult and not a small child either.

If you have any African themed meals please send them in for next week to neverseconds@gmail.com along with any questions for Malawi!

Mutsale bwino! (Good bye in Chichewa.)

Veg

Saturday 29th September

"No I won't. I will not."

Martha was doing all she could to avoid looking into £42,000 worth of BBC camera that was balanced on the back of the airline seat in front of her. Watching her reflection in the big lens I noted the effects of the previous 24 hours of travelling. After an overnight flight from London we'd met Laura and Ray, the BBC documentary team, in Johannesburg and together we were sharing the last hop to Blantyre in southern Malawi. The plane was packed and everyone's attention was on the camera and where it was pointing.

"No worries Martha," Ray the cameraman said moving the huge camera to the side.

BBC Scotland had approached Mary's Meals with the idea to make a programme about the blog and Martha's journey to Lirangwe School, and so it was that Martha found herself at 35,000ft with only a few hours sleep expressing her nervous excitement by refusing to cooperate. We'd already met Ray and Laura at home in Lochgilphead for a day of filming and getting to know each other, and it had been clear immediately that Martha felt uncomfortable on camera. But when distracted by building a model Malawian village house she'd chatted away contentedly oblivious to the camera, and so pens, paper and diaries were packed for the trip. We hoped the coverage on TV and in the press would raise Mary's Meals' profile but in order to do it we had to put ourselves in front of the cameras. Martha found it hardest to do and her unease struck me as she looked across the aisle at me.

"Come on Martha. Just do the simple things simply and we'll all help you do the hard things," I said. The family and crew

could support her in every way but we couldn't smile for her or talk for her. Being the centre of attention seemed to be the problem. Blending in at school was a skill that she had come to rely on with the recent difficulties. Putting your head above any parapet attracts attention from all sides yet for the next four days the focus of the camera would return time and time again to her. Watching her struggle on the plane the enormity of the trip began to sink in. The 5600 miles that slipped away underneath us were the easy part of the journey. Immunisation injections and packing were already forgotten but I felt woefully unprepared for the emotional journey we were beginning or for how we would support Martha through it.

Smaller than England, Malawi was a long thin country south of the equator and the famous Lake Malawi took up 20% of country. Densely populated with over 15 million people, who lived mainly in rural areas as subsistence farmers, it was one of the poorest countries in the world. A rapidly expanding population and the failure of the rains to come had resulted in lack of food, particularly in the south where Blantyre was situated.

Filming with a documentary team is part fly on the wall and part acting. We were becoming used to requests to do bizarre things for the camera and after a dozen or so rides up and down the escalator in Edinburgh Airport a simple trot back up the steps to remerge from the plane on the Blantyre tarmac was easily done. Flushed from the heat and the embarrassment of parading we were distracted from taking in the sights in front of us. Beyond the plane scrub extended away in shades of dry brown until it met a solitary tree on the horizon. Daylight hours had little variation in Malawi throughout the year and so seasons, as we understood them, didn't exist. We were at the end of the dry season and expectations were high for the November rains. Crisp dry leaves tinkled as they blew across the ground and it was odd to have one of the sounds of autumn in the heat of a Malawian day.

The airport building was tiny and chaotic as bags waited on the carousel for flustered travellers to retrieve. Mary's Meals' staff met us on the other side of immigration and with a nod from customs we were off. At the exit a crowd of men, kept at bay by a uniformed official, jostled for position eager to help

carry our bags for a few Kwatcha. The official barked a few words of Chichewa at them and a gap just large enough to squeeze through appeared. Polly, fearless as ever, lunged through it. We all followed and our reluctance to let go of our bags was graciously accepted by the eager porters. Fears from the BBC that there would be press awaiting us were unfounded and following the light blue Mary's Meals t-shirted staff member we reached our minibus.

"You ok kids?" I asked, looking at each in turn.

Joe looked most frazzled. Sleep had come hardest to him overnight. Polly clutched Fingal, her teddy, close to her and Martha had her bag of books at her feet. The girls had brought tangible homely items with them but Joe, whose greatest comfort was the familiarity of a computer, had no such luck.

"It's too hot," he said.

Gazing at the Orion constellation over the tip of the wing all night he'd proved he was old enough to keep himself awake whilst still being too young for coffee.

"Look! Look!" Martha called in excitement. Across the road as we pulled away was a lady with a large dish on her head.

"She's using no hands!" Polly added in wonderment, craning to stare at the beautifully balanced walker for as long as she could.

Each twist in the road revealed new sights which were to become familiar. Bricks were made where needed and large neat stacks adjoined the roadside. Each stack had passageways at the bottom so wood could be burnt to fire the bricks. Buildings seemed to be either going up or falling down and small wooden shelters lined the road. We stopped at one and we all got out for a look. People began to appear from all directions as Ray hoisted the camera to his shoulder. Approaching the stall we could see that it was a stainless steel worktop with a large circular dent beaten into it. Under the make shift fryer a wood fire burned, sizzling the oil as handfuls of peeled Irish potatoes, as they called them, were thrown in. As Martha and I posed for photos a voice from the back called, "Don't eat them! They could be fried in cooling oil!" Smiling politely Martha and I put down the chips.

"Zikomo kwambiri," I offered our thanks in Chichewa as

a member of the Mary's Meals staff first gave the stall holder something for his time then explained to us that people stole the oil from electricity transformers to cook with. Something as familiar and as simple as a chip had taught us our first real-life lesson about Malawi.

Meeting the Mary's Meals Country Director for Malawi that afternoon, the enormity of the task the charity had under taken was made clear. Feeding 550,000 primary school children daily across Malawi represented just 20% of the school roll. When Mary's Meals expanded into a new school the immediate effect was the number of children attending school increased and exam results improved. Women from surrounding villages keen to improve the chances for their children took it in turns to arrive at the school at 5am to start making the Likuni Phala, the porridge Mary's Meals serves. Once a month different coloured bags of porridge were delivered and monitors from Mary's Meals headquarters travelled around the schools by motorbike checking there were enough pots to cook in and enough porridge to meet the demands of the school. The numbers danced over Martha's head as John, Rebecca and I listened to the breakdown of the operation and tried to comprehend the figures.

"Did you understand it, Martha?" I asked after the Director had left.

"Yeah, Dad. There are starving kids not in school and Mary's Meals does something about it."

Martha Payne and David Payne

NeverSeconds One primary school pupil's daily dose of school dinners.

SATURDAY, 29 SEPTEMBER 2012

Arriving Malawi

When I got on the South African Airways plane at
Heathrow to fly to Johannesburg I was very excited.
I sat next to my brother and I could look out of the
window. On the back of the seat in front of me was a
screen and I could see how far we had to travel.

I had earphones and could watch the plane from a camera
on the tail fin and it was the best take off ever. The
stewards brought us our dinner and we had a choice. I
chose the lamb.

It was very tasty and I visited the kitchen to see how
they make it. The steward said they heat it dry or with
steam. They also recycle lots of things including the foil
lid and cup. They are a good airline for recycling. There
were lots of dishes including a dessert and the cheese
and biscuits were very good. I ate everything apart from

the roll which I gave to dad.

Food-o-meter- 8/10
Mouthfuls- I was far too excited to count
Health Rating- 9/10
Pieces of hair- 0

It was hard to sleep on the plane because the people behind us had their lights on all through the night. I managed to sleep a wee bit but I was very tired. We woke up early and had breakfast before landing at Johannesburg.

It was quite cold in Johannesburg and we met Ray and Laura from the BBC at the airport. We played cards because the flight was delayed.

It was hot in Blantyre and I lay down on the marble floor to get cool. My chinchilla has a marble slab for the same reason.

Blantyre airport is very small and they use a tractor to pull the baggage carts. It was a massey ferguson and dad was excited about it. There were lots of porters waiting to carry our bags and it was very noisy as we left the airport.

We stopped at a stall on the way to where we were staying. There was a lovely toddler on his mum's knee. He held my hand for a second and then got shy. Lots of children my age have babies wrapped up in material slung across their backs and it looks really heavy. None of the babies cry. There are no pavements and even children walk along the road. There are people walking everywhere. I spotted 5 Mary's Meals shelters on the way to where we are staying. It got dark very quickly and Mum made me put on insect repellent which tastes bitter if you get it in your mouth. If I roll over at night a mosquito may bite me through the net. I am going to sleep right in the middle of my bed.

Sunday 30th September

Bumping along a dust road at 6am wasn't how most people began their day in Malawi. Although light, the sun hadn't cleared the surrounding hills and in the half dawn we passed people already going about their daily business. Carved into the hillside were areas that had been cleared and planted. Narrow terraces had been cut on the steeper ground and despite the early hour were already being worked. The rains hadn't come last year and so no harvest had been made in the south of Malawi. Many of the people walking along the track had a sack of government issue maize balanced on their heads, ready to be pounded, winnowed and finally milled into flour. Only then could it be mixed with water and cooked into a paste the colour and texture of mashed potato. Nsima was the staple food and often eaten with beans as the main meal. Our little convoy pulled to a halt as the sun finally cleared the hill and in the growing light we could see a collection of half a dozen brick and mud huts set back from the road.

"Is this where he lives, Dad?" Martha asked from the rear seat of the minibus.

She was referring to Ben, a boy of her age whom Mary's Meals had arranged for us to meet and share a day with.

"Must be."

Martha pressed her nose against the glass and looked along the footpath towards the houses.

"Will he like me, Dad?"

"Of course he will. Help him with his chores and show him your photos. It'll be amazing and we're all here to help."

Holding the photos Martha allowed herself to be threaded with the microphone and set off towards the village followed

by the cameras.

Ben stood with his mum and brother, Abel, by the entrance to their house. Smaller than Martha, he was bare footed in shorts and a shirt and he greeted Martha with a smile as nervous as hers. He led Martha around the side of the house to where grass matting had been placed upon the ground beside a sheet of sewn together maize bags. With a translator from Mary's Meals they sat together on the raised plinth of the house under the overhanging eaves of the thatched roof. Unsure whether to look at each other or the translator when talking, Martha and Ben started to exchange a few words and soon the photographs were out and Martha was reenacting an epic snowball fight whilst showing Ben a picture of our sheep in the snow. Turning the next photo to reveal a picture of our house, Martha shuffled it to the back again immediately. Ben's home was square with sides about three metres long. Inside it was dark. There were no windows and the space was split into three areas, one for pots and pans, one for the kids to sleep and one for their mum to sleep. There was neither furniture nor decoration and Ben, like the rest of his family, slept on the compacted soil floor. There was no electricity or lights and so no chance for Ben and his mum to read or work after sundown. Martha was distracted by howls of laughter from around the corner. Women and children had gathered and were sat playing with Rebecca and Polly. Polly was touching a young girl's hair who in turn stroked hers. The ladies did the same and soon everyone was laughing at the differences.

All the kids joined together in their fascination with the cameras. Joe and Polly were taking photos of the kids and showing them the results but neither could compete with the BBC's huge camera and soon Ray was teaching the kids how to film each other as they struck poses in front of the lens. The awkwardness of descending on their village was gone in the melee of kids playing and to the soundtrack of laughter Martha and Ben set off for water.

The eroded footpath went downhill steeply and boulders and roots crossed the route. Ben led the way with Martha following along. Dust kicked up from their feet helped track their progress down to the stream bed, which they crossed to climb

the hill beyond. Swinging a large metal pail by his side Ben knew every foot placement from the countless occasions he used this route and after sometime they reached the borehole. The metal pump's long arm needed working hard to raise the water and side by side Martha and Ben worked to fill the pail. Each action threw a handful of clear water out and slowly the pail was filled. Casually, with Abel's help, Ben raised the bucket to his head and set off along the track home. Not to be outdone, Martha took a smaller plastic bucket, filled it, and set off after Ben. Not a dropped was spilled by Ben whilst Martha's inexperienced steps caused water to slosh over and wet her. Unable to watch any more Abel took the bucket from Martha and I took the bucket pail from Ben. I couldn't walk alongside the wee lad just watching as he carried what felt like 25kgs of water on his head without helping. Getting it on my head I felt the bottom of the pail flex and then with slow steps and a steadying hand I crossed the burn and climbed the hill to his house. It was hard and in the growing heat I struggled.

There was no breakfast for Ben back at his house. Martha threw me a worried glance. Despite her early breakfast the heat and effort of collecting water was already more than Martha was used to. Watching the two of them set off for school reminded me of her first day at Lochgilphead Primary School. Familiar with the school grounds from dropping off and picking up Joe, she had shot me one backwards glance before disappearing in line through the double doors. Here in the dust she did the same but she lingered and held my gaze for a fraction longer than was comfortable. The style of filming for the documentary required the camera to encroach on Martha's comfort zone. She was hanging on by a thread but determined not to disappoint. The pressure she was under wasn't being shaken off with the natural exuberance of a nine year old, it was stressing her in the same way it would an adult and I feared the journey of a lifetime would not become the cherished memory for her we had hoped.

Nipping ahead in the minibus we waited for the two of them to arrive. Right on cue as they broached the final hill first a chicken and then a goat crossed the path in front of them to complete the Malawian scene. Nankofi Number One was a school of 400 of which a quarter were in Standard One, the first

class children attend when starting school at age six. If there was any doubt of the child's age they were asked to reach over their head with their arm and touch their ear on the opposite side. Success meant a place at school and a Mary's Meal but failure meant a wait for the next enrolment session.

The classrooms were brick with concrete floors and a tin roof. Even at 7.30am they were beginning to get warm and with more than a 100 children per room the conditions would be stifling despite the unglazed windows. The news of a film crew had spread and a crowd was gathering as Ben and Martha approached. Rebecca was talking mum to mum and introducing her children. Local mums took pride in sharing theirs. Loveness, Peace, Memory and Hope were cuddled and on her arrival Martha was being taught clapping games. It was a scene familiar to playgrounds across the world and language was no barrier to the grimaces and smiles as claps were forgotten and rhythms refound. Joe produced the football we had brought as a gift for Ben and instigated a Scotland v Malawi international. Outnumbered and out skilled, he relied on his size and stout footwear against bare feet to force one goal through the make shift posts and the crowd went wild. All the kids were enjoying themselves and in amongst them somewhere were my three.

"You must smile. You must, you must."

Grabbing my hand was a young man with a suit jacket over his polo shirt.

"I am Michaels. Headmaster. You must smile. Mary's Meals does this."

I thought I had been smiling but compared to the broad grins that were surrounding us I needed to try harder.

"Your school children look very happy, Michaels."

"My learners are happy. They have Mary's Meals. They learn now. Yes we are happy."

Letting go of my hand to point at the children, Michaels nodded to me.

"Yes, you must smile like them."

Tired and dusty, Martha leaned into me in the minibus on the way home.

"Ben was cool, Dad. He was so funny with his games."

"I liked his mum. She was very proud of her boys and it was nice Grandpa John got to meet Ben's grandparents as well."

"Agogo John," Martha called over to John in the bus. "Agogo is Chichewa for grandparent. I'm going to call Grandpa Agogo John instead now."

John smiled back. We had connected with Ben's family across all the generations and the love and effort both families went to for their children was apparent. Ben's school dinner debate was about having something to eat at all and ours was about the quality of the food we served our children. We certainly had things to learn from each other.

Martha Payne and David Payne

NeverSeconds One primary school pupil's daily dose of school dinners.

SUNDAY, 30 SEPTEMBER 2012

Meeting Ben and his family

I didn't mind getting up early to meet Ben. Ben is my age and lives in a nearby village with no roads or electricity. He gets up and starts his jobs when it is light and I was going to meet him.

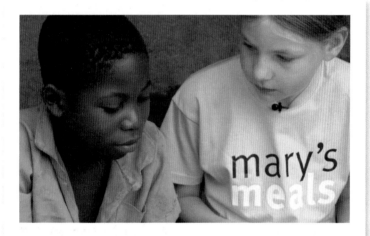

His house is square with 3 metre long sides. The thatched roof comes very low and we sat under it to chat. Florian from Mary's Meals translated for us. Ben liked my photos from home. He doesn't understand snow because he has never seen it. He liked my sheep and hens though. Ben didn't have any toys but his friends had a car made out of a milk bottle. I have never met anyone with no toys.

Ben has to help his mum with jobs if he is not at school. I went with him to fetch water. The pump is a long way away and Ben carries the water home on his head. I tried to carry a small bucket home and I got very wet.

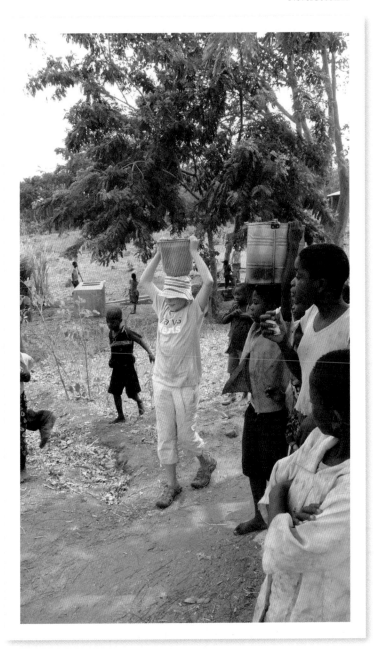

Dad helped Ben with his bucket and said it was very difficult. Once we got the water to Ben's house it was time to go to school. Ben doesn't wear shoes and he is much faster than me walking also. It wasn't hot yet because it was still very early. It was hard to keep up with Ben up the hills. I spotted the school in the distance. I didn't realise what it was because it is just a few buildings. There is no sign and the classrooms have no doors or windows. Inside there are plastic benches to sit on given by the last president. They are the colour of his political party.

Ben likes school and wants to be a doctor. I told him Mum is a doctor and he thought that was lucky for me so that I always had the right medicines. Primary school is free in Malawi and you must pass a written exam to get into the next year. Classes have lots of different ages because of this. Ben gets a Mary's Meal every day and he showed me his mug. He likes the likuni phala because it gives him enough energy to study well. I was hungry at Ben's school after getting water and walking there even though I had a breakfast. Ben's family only have enough food for an evening meal and so he gets nothing before school.

I played lots of games in the playground with all the children that came. I learnt new skipping games and new clapping games.

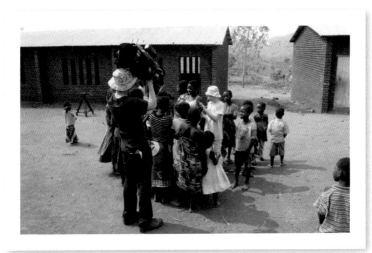

I gave Ben a football from Scotland. We had a lot of fun playing catch. He tricked me by looking at his brother but throwing the ball to me. Ben was so happy I forgot he was hungry. I don't think Ben forgets.

Monday 1st October

For me it was the water jug. Rebecca seemed to have chosen the coffee pot and Agogo John was concentrating on the foliage of a young tree visible through the window. Anything was preferable to looking at each other. Each of us was only just coping with our emotions and even a glance would have been enough to cause breakdown. This was just another day in Martha's emotional world but to an Argyll smallholder, a doctor and a Mary's Meals volunteer less used to embracing our softer sides the day ahead was more challenging. More than 7000 people had chosen to put their hands in their pockets and donate to fund the kitchen. I wanted a joyous day for them. A day celebrating the positive power of the internet that had protected Martha from the council cronies and brought from the depth of despair a great coming together of support for hungry children without school dinners. The kids at Lirangwe didn't need our tears they needed our support. I wished the TV camera had a confidence filter so that my awkward emotional self would be seen by the viewers as a smiling dad able to join in with the celebrations with a smile, clap or dance. The kids had no such issues. Joe was looking forward to some maths lessons, hopefully in Standard 7 and Polly was keen to help the Standard 1's with their phala. Painting the sign was Martha's focus. Subsequently breakfast was dominated by children's chatter and there was no silence to allow us adults to further wallow in our thoughts.

We'd been invited to arrive at the school just after the 7.30am assembly. Briefed in the minibus as we travelled through Blantyre we were made aware that many of the children would have eaten little over the weekend and some would have eaten nothing. Rebecca had spotted some signs of malnutrition in

the children at Ben's school. A pot belly and a reddish tinge to the hair were the easiest to identify but eye infections and sores were also common. HIV/AIDS was responsible for a lot of deaths amongst adults and had left some children at Lirangwe orphaned and homeless. We encouraged the kids to shake everyone's hands but not to put their fingers in their mouths and to wash and then gel their hands before eating. Dirty clothes were not a sign of poverty. Within minutes of walking in the dust our clean clothes were tinged and once you began sitting in classes or leaning against buildings it became worse. In Mary's Meals t-shirts we all bounced along the dirt road to the school. The press had gone ahead and I recognised their van as we swung into the school yard.

We heard them immediately even above the idling engine of the minibus. 2000 children were in full song. The unmistakable lilt and rhythm of Africa took away all resolve we had struggled to muster. The power of the song increased as Ray opened the minibus door to greet us. Raising his voice to be heard he told us not to worry.

"We're all doing it," he said, gesturing with a screwed up fist at his eyes. It was a kind thing to say and I felt less embarrassed at the struggle I was facing with my tears.

"Are you ready, Martha?" asked Florian from Mary's Meals. She nodded and gripped my hand.

The children were lined up in classes with their teachers. Each line was more than a hundred strong and snaked from the raised walkway from which a teacher was directing the singing. Faces turned to us as we walked alongside the line of oldest children to the steps up to the walkway. With a switch of his cane the conductor indicated a change of song and voices in unison sang:

"We are happy today, we are happy today..."

Walking along until we were in the middle we were unsure what to do next. Martha was finding it hard to face the singers whose voices we were now as much feeling as hearing. Down on one knee I gave her as much encouragement as I could.

"Don't be scared love. They're just happy you are here."

"Are they filming me?"

"I'm not sure. Ray's probably getting footage of the kids

singing."

She could see the tears in my eyes and gave my hand an extra squeeze. It should have been me giving her strength but I took some of hers gratefully. Martha did not see herself as any sort of hero deserving of song and the praise directed to her was difficult for her young years to comprehend. There was no one else the Lirangwe children could thank though and so as the song changed again I jumped down amongst the kids and beckoned Martha to follow.

"Let's go say hi. Come on, Martha!"

She leaned forward into my arms and we began by walking down the lines of youngest children. Their shyness gave way to smiles as we greeted them in Chichewa.

"Muli bwanji. Muli Bwanje."

We weaved our way down lines trying to thank as many children as possible for their kind and amazing welcome. I felt my phone buzz in my pocket.

"Hello. I can't hear you we're at Lirangwe and the kids are singing. You'll need to shout."

"It's BBC Radio 4 Today programme here. Can we talk to Martha? ...Hello? ...Mr Payne?"

It was incredible that Today was interested but all I could do was hold the phone high and hope they were recording the rejoicing voices. Slowly the pressure of tears was easing and out of the blur individual faces were becoming clearer. The generosity of many wasn't being squandered by Mary's Meals. The efficiency of the charity ensured that the money ended up as porridge in the stomachs of children. Every development outcome for these children had been improved by the simple addition of a Mary's Meal to their school day and they seemed to know it.

We were led to the headmistress's office where, out of the camera's eye, we had a moment to sit. Rebecca and John looked as blown away as I felt and from the red eyes I had not been the only one to shed a tear. Polly was smiling having enjoyed every moment and Joe too seemed buoyed up by the experience.

"Did you hear them?" he asked. "They were singing your name, Martha. All of them. I mean every single one of them was singing it. That's awesome."

"It's embarrassing," she said, raising a smile.

Rebecca reached over and gave her a huge hug.

"Mind the microphone!" she teased her mum.

"Listen to the TV star!" Rebecca answered without easing off and Martha folded into her lap. Nine was an incredible age to make a difference but still not too old to be comforted with a cuddle from her mum.

The headmistress entered and on instinct we all sat more upright and Martha took back her own chair. Her thanks were no less effusive than the children's. She explained how the rainy season would be upon them soon and how the old wood and thatched shelter would not have coped. Children would have been without phala and they would have stopped coming to school. A break in their education would set them back when it came to exams. There were too many children for the class-rooms and so the old kitchen was now used as a classroom and the kitchen shelter served as another in the afternoon. As we were chatting the children returned to class and the singing gave way to the bustling noise of a busy school. Children moved in groups towards class and were persuaded to do so quickly by stick-wielding teachers who flicked purposefully at their heels. Some learners had books with them carried in old bread bags or folded into a cardboard square bound with twisted carrier bags. Drifting from the kitchen was the tantalising nutty aroma of cooking likuni phala. As the children passed near their heads turned towards the source and I could see how eagerly awaited it was.

"Can I see it now?" Martha asked hopefully, pointing in the direction of the kitchen. A nod indicated the media were in position and so with more deep breaths we set off. The school yard hidden under the feet of the learners was revealed to be strewn with boulders and bricks and it took some care to approach the kitchen without tripping. The nutty smell grew stronger and the cooks grew strong in voice as they took oppor-tunity to welcome Martha to the kitchen. High on the outside wall was the unfinished painted sign:

Mary's Meals Centre – Lirangwe
"Kindly donated by Friends of ------------"

Inside, six pots on top of efficient wood burning rocket stoves were being stirred with long wooden staffs. Each pot heated 150 litres of water mixed with one 20kg sack of likuni phala to produce enough for 300-350 children. At first light the dinner ladies had carried the water from the bore hole 200 metres away in drums on their heads. Three hours later and the thick porridge was approaching readiness. The dinner ladies sang and danced resplendent in their Mary's Meals chitenjes. The wrap around skirt material printed with a design of porridge stirring ladies was highly valued by the cooks as part of volunteering. As they stirred Rebecca and John took turns to help. Back in a less daunting situation we were able to enjoy the occasion and Rebecca was into the swing of it with hips moving in time to the rhythm of the song. The fires were hot and concern was expressed for Martha moving amongst them. She was nervous being so close but gave stirring a go. The texture of the porridge was thick and it was an effort to keep the porridge moving to prevent sticking.

Encouraged by the singing ladies the artist, who was waiting patiently next to the sign outside, offered Martha a brush and some paint. Taking them both she climbed the sand pile to the sign.

Outlined in faint pencil was the word NeverSeconds for her to finish. Despite being up above us and with the dinner ladies singing and stamping beneath her, Martha found calm in the task. She seemed to close her mind to the unusual things going on around her and tested the sweep of the brush on the back of her hand before dipping it gently into the pot of blue paint. Dabbing the excess off onto the rim she scrunched up her face in concentration and lay a clear stroke of paint down the letter 'N'. Not looking for approval and confident in her own ability she returned the brush to the pot and continued. She had looked forward to this moment for so long that to see her enjoying every stroke of the brush was wonderful. With uncharacteristic exuberance I whooped, cheered and shouted my praise up to her.

"It's looking great, Martha. Well done!"

There was so much noise she might not have heard me but she didn't need to. The practiced care and attention she had

given every blog post was being demonstrated in her approach to painting the sign. She was back on familiar ground and loving it. Oblivious to Ray's filming and the staccato clicking of camera shutters Martha finished the 'N' and continued. Painting the sign had been what she had wanted to come and enjoy and she was savouring the moment. With help from Joe and Polly she finished the sign, which signalled the next round of celebrations. The school choir had gathered beneath her and they launched into voice. Stood high above them she listened as songs about her were sung and a small play acted out. From her expression I could not tell her thoughts but she couldn't stop glancing back at the sign, smiling each time.

Getting the phala from six cooking pots into the stomachs of 2000 children was a practiced routine at Lirangwe and women in pairs filled large plastic drums from the pots then carried them to outside the classes. Children queued with their plastic mugs that had been given to them when they started school by Mary's Meals. Martha helped pour each child a measured amount of phala from a jug straight into their mugs. Full mugs were held carefully with a reverence and carried to a favourite shady spot. Some children had spoons; others took leaves from trees or just used a blade of grass to scoop the thick phala into their mouths. Across the school children were starting to eat and calmness descended. The background noise of chattering children was replaced with the soft sound of porridge eating. I'd expected hungry children to eat quickly but it was explained that their small stomachs filled easily and that they needed time to eat it all. I could see some children spooning porridge into bags to take home for siblings or parents. The phala was sustaining whole families and to see a hungry child put their needs second to help another was heartbreaking. First from one corner of the yard and then from another the rough sound of scrapping started. Phala was being finished and every last morsel was being chased around the mug until it could be removed and eaten. It wasn't the quick lucky swirl of a teaspoon around a yoghurt pot but a slow deliberate seeking of every last grain of nourishment. Watching the children's faces you could tell the exact moment when they resigned themselves to accepting there was no more. Heads dropped slightly and eyes

rose from the mugs to look around. Chatter began to pick up and then movement as friends found each other again.

Martha had finished serving duties and was sat with a class eating her own mug of phala.

"You can taste the wood smoke. It's crunchy in places and it's really filling. I like it. Try it, Dad."

She handed me her mug and spoon. The phala was the colour of a sandy beach and thick enough to hold the spoon in the middle. I'd learnt from watching the other children that it would be hot and cautiously I tried a cooled spoonful from the edge. The flavour had an earthy nuttiness to it.

"Will you rate it?" I asked her.

"10 out of 10 food-o-meter definitely and the same health rating. I forgot to count my mouthfuls and no hair. It's perfect!"

High praise indeed and looking at the children of Lirangwe who could argue.

MONDAY, 1 OCTOBER 2012

Lirangwe- Friends of NeverSeconds

I didn't sleep well because the fan in my room is noisy. It is nice to be cool but I may turn the fan off because it kept me awake. I was very nervous in the van going to Lirangwe. I was shaking with nerves. When we got there all the children were lined up singing and I could hear them over the sound of the van engine.

When we got out and stood in front of them you could feel the song in your chest. Dad, Mum and Grandpa all had wet eyes and I had to squeeze dad's hand. It was a nice song and I went down to the children to thank them. I said 'Muli bwanji' which means 'hello how are you' and 'Zikomo kwambiri' which means 'thank you'. After we had said hello properly we went to the headmistress's office. Joe spotted a wad of papers pinned to the wall. It was the school Death Record and it was very thick.

Next we went to the kitchen to meet the ladies making the likuni phala. They were very happy and danced.

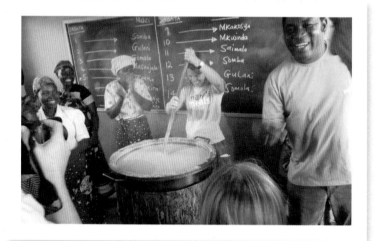

There were 6 massive pots of porridge being cooked and the ladies were singing as they stirred it. One lady had her baby strapped to her back but he didn't wake up. I had a go at stirring but I got smoke in my eyes from the wood fire because I am short. The pots were massive and I think I could have had a bath in one. The sign had been left for me to complete and there was a sand pile for me to stand on.

I liked the colour of blue I used to finish the sign. It's my favourite. I was very careful about doing it and I almost used too much but the artist helped me. I hope you like our sign. I tried my best and Joe and Polly helped.

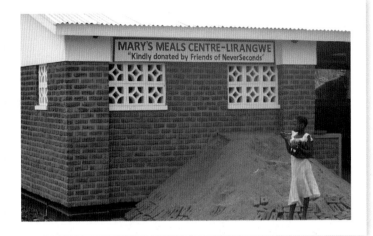

I helped serve out the phala to the children. I used a jug to give everyone the same.

Some children didn't eat all their porridge so they could take it home to their family to share. I find it hard not to eat when I am hungry and it is one of the bravest things I have ever seen.

I had some phala with an older class. One boy in the class was called Gilbert and he had sent me a message through Mary's Meals. Gilbert's an orphan. His dad was eaten by a crocodile and Gilbert lives in the market at night on his own.

Gilbert wants to be president when he grows up and he said he would make sure no child will be hungry in Malawi. Gilbert for president!

Martha Payne and David Payne

We all made lots of friends. Here is Polly's friend. They
stayed together all day.

Everyone is very proud of the kitchen at the school and
so am I.

Tuesday 2nd October

Martha had fussed over her backpack for weeks back home. The clothing items had been changed. A packet of colouring pencils swapped for felt tips and a plain paper pad, for sketching, had been placed alongside the lined notebook for school work. A couple of pencils and pens, a rubber, ruler and pencil sharpener completed the pencil case. Wrapped in a towel were a bar of soap, toothpaste and a toothbrush. Finally a tennis ball was added for fun. It wasn't the first backpack she had donated to Mary's Meals but she was going to share this backpack personally, as were Joe and Polly. Mindful of the BBC I'd chosen three brightly coloured plain bags which were easy for the camera to spot.

Our bags came out with us but for the rest the journey had taken more time. Back in the UK school classes often got involved in the backpack scheme and a Mary's Meals volunteer would start the process with a talk in the school. Returning to collect the backpacks sometime later, the bags' journey would then start. Each backpack, labelled to indicate if it was for a boy or girl and for what age group, was collected by the Mary's Meals van and transported to Glasgow. Backpacks were packed into large white sacks and when sufficient numbers were collected a shipping container was delivered and volunteers filled the container. The delivery we were about to distribute had left Glasgow on Thursday 14th June and was sent on its way by Colin Jackson. Travelling via the port of Beira in Mozambique then overland to Blantyre, Malawi, its journey time could have varied mainly due to whether there were any fuel shortages for the lorry.

Mary's Meals had to be fair to the schools it supported and

schools were given backpacks in order. When preparing for a distribution steps were taken to ensure the day passed smoothly. Schools were not informed until moments before the lorry arrived and the distribution aimed to be done within a couple of hours before large crowds could gather and disrupt the process.

Waking the kids early again I was glad our time with the BBC was ending today. It had brought more strain to the trip than we could ever have imagined. The simple act of observing us was changing the way we were behaving. All of us worried about saying or doing something wrong that the cameras would capture. The trust we had with Ray and Laura was above reproach and the fears existed solely in our heads but it was our heads that were being played with most by what we were seeing. The compression of all we had experienced into a few days had left us exhausted and without energy to process the events we had witnessed. We were receiving text messages from friends saying that they had seen footage back home and that it was fantastic. Between the newspapers, Real Radio and the BBC the audience for our adventure was huge. News items had been translated into six languages for the global BBC audience and footage was being broadcast on BBC World News. We had no idea who was watching the coverage but if the impact on the viewer was even a fraction of the impact on us then the effect would be extraordinary.

"Morning girls," I attempted in my cheeriest 5am wakeup call voice. Both were flat out and needed gentle shaking to be brought to.

"Backpacks today," I encouraged them. It seemed to have the desired effect and legs swung down under the nets and tired eyes were rubbed into use.

We made quite a sight at the breakfast table. With children sat between adults long arms were passing around the cereal and coaxing the little ones into eating. We still had not discussed the day at Lirangwe between us and now was not the time either. Shock was still the overwhelming emotion and until that feeling subsided we were unable to begin reflecting on the day's events with any effectiveness. Lirangwe was boxed away in each of our heads safely but today was another day and I was proud the kids were looking forward to it as much as we were.

The focus for the cameras would be the backpacks, each lovingly packed and sent on its way by a person back home, and not us. Helping share the kind gifts of others was an honour we were looking forward to.

"Never had a gift. Can you imagine that?" I thought out loud.

"Like Charlie Bucket?" Polly asked.

"Charlie had a chocolate bar every year, Polly," Martha was pleased to know.

"Not Christmas or birthdays?" Joe quizzed.

"I don't think so. These backpacks are going to be amazing for these kids. I'm not sure I can imagine how it would feel to be given your first gift."

"Let's go find out then!" Joe grinned, swinging an arm in affirmation and by chance the toot of a car horn indicated we were due to go. Perfect comic timing and enough to replace tired looks with big smiles all round.

"Dad!" Martha shouted, pointing a warning finger at the lorry driving ahead. It was lurching from side to side trying to find the easiest route along the worn dirt road. The angle of lean it reached seemed to defy gravity but each time it righted itself slowly and we continued to make progress. A Mary's Meals pickup had gone ahead five minutes before with the good news and we were expecting to arrive and find all the children in their classrooms waiting.

Pulling up in the centre of the large courtyard, our every move was watched by faces pressed against the decorative concrete air blocks that took the place of windows. The children were in class and knew why we were here. An excited hum was coming from the rooms. There was no time to dawdle and the Mary's Meals staff had the lorry open and white sacks of backpacks were manhandled to the classes. I followed Joe to a class, dragging a white sack with me. Inside, over a hundred children were waiting, wide eyed and expectant. Organised into two queues, one for boys and one for girls, Joe and I started handing backpacks out. Mary's Meals staff had checked each backpack at the warehouse in Blantyre to ensure they were as equitable as possible. Heavy and tightly packed it was hard to free each individual backpack but as soon as we managed a pair

of hands appeared to receive the gift. Watching the children return to their spot in the classroom with backpacks wrapped up in their arms we could see they didn't quite believe it. No one was allowed to open their bags until the whole class had received theirs and the children were incredibly patient. Finally each child had a backpack and was seated. The Mary's Meals volunteer told the children in Chichewa how people in the UK and packed these bags and sent them over as gifts. On the count of three permission was to be given to open them and Joe made the count as loud as he could.

"One…" Bags were on knees.

"Two…" Zips were located.

"Three…" A moment of mass unzipping was followed by a shared gasp, a millisecond's silent pause as the eyes took in the delights and then a roar of happiness began. Each discovery drove the roar louder and pens and pencils were held overhead and flapped in joy like sporting trophies at a final. Towels were unrolled and wrapped around shoulders and the soft material tested on cheeks. Notebooks, each a week's wages in Malawi, were championed and pens tested neatly on back pages. The likuni phala brought the energy to the classroom to learn and the backpacks were bringing the tools. The roar was not subsiding and the teacher moved amongst the kids acknowledging them as they showed her the contents from their backpacks. Smiles abounded and Joe and I slipped away to the next class. Back in the open air we could hear the same results from different classrooms and spotting the journalists we found Martha doing exactly the same in another class. There were smiles, the roar and the appreciation from the kids. There was more to these backpacks than just the sum of their contents. They were giving each and every child a message. A message that they were not forgotten and that children across the UK were thinking of them. From thousands of miles away a child's hope was being sent and accepted with gratitude.

NeverSeconds **One primary school pupil's daily dose of school dinners.**

TUESDAY, 2 OCTOBER 2012

Backpacks, Ntenjera Primary School

This is William loading the truck at the Mary's Meals warehouse in Blantyre.

We bounced all the way to Ntenjera Primary School. I thought the lorry might fall over onto a man on a bike but it didn't. No one at the school knew the backpacks were coming and so all the children were in their classrooms with their teachers. When the children saw the lorry they knew it was full of backpacks and I could hear how excited they were.

The children queued up and I handed them each a backpack. Some classes had more than a 150 children in. It was great fun because they were all so happy. When all the children had a backpack I counted to three and they opened them. Everyone seemed to like the pens best.

There was a big queue of girls waiting to get backpacks. It took a long time to hand out all 1960 backpacks and it was very hot in the classrooms but some children sat on bricks outside. I gave my backpack to Christina who was older than me but the same size. It's hard to tell how old children are because they grow up hungry and they are smaller but older than me. All the kids loved their backpacks and I am going to send more.

When I had an interview with Laura I took a photo of Ray
so you can see what it is like to talk to a camera all day!

Martha Payne and David Payne

The Future

Travelling to Lirangwe I had spotted a huge neat painted bill-board for a local bolt manufacturer. 'Any bolt replaced' it read. Feelings unfortunately aren't like broken bolts. Bolts are easily defined by thread type, length, metal and head. A broken bolt was easily replaced and apart from a newish sheen to the part no one would be the wiser. Some of my emotions were seized from lack of use and I struggled to name them let alone replace them with shiny working ones. I wasn't practiced in discussing my feelings and the words to describe them did not readily spring to mind. It wasn't just me. Each of us had struggled in our final interviews with the BBC. More formally set out than anything we had done before, we'd all been encouraged by Laura's smile to give our all in our responses. There were moments from our time in Malawi that I had stashed in my head like a photo in Martha's album. Images that I needed to hold onto until I'd learnt the language to discuss them. Some of the emotions that I'd had cause to practice from the outset of NeverSeconds were the wrong ones to have brought to Malawi.

My anger and frustration with Argyll and Bute council was not being soothed by time. Thinly veiled attacks on our parenting on national radio and an abusive phone call stood out as examples of a public body sick to the very top. Complaints via the proper procedures and through elected councillors had brought no visible changes. Far from being contrite about their actions they seemed to take a pride in being untouchable. I could only hope that the political embarrassment the council had brought upon itself was enough to spur action at government level to sort them out. Martha seemed to have put it behind her and wrote in The Sunday Times:

'I don't feel upset about the ban now because it has helped raise so much money for Mary's Meals.'

Forgiving is a mainstay of playground friendships and seeing Martha extend the same to the council made their lack of apology even more grating. She had brought her propensity for sharing in the playground to sharing on her blog. From the days of sharing her dinner it had grown to a place where children from around the world had shared theirs. A food blogger at heart she had moulded NeverSeconds into a blog about food issues for children and one of those issues was that some children did not have enough. Balanced with her scores for her own dinners was an acknowledgement that she was privileged. She had taken to heart the advice I had received from my Argyll farming friend, 'Doesn't matter who you help, just help someone,' and she had done just that. Beyond the fundraising that stood at £120,000 she had done something maybe more powerful. She had demonstrated why children deserve the rights they have.

My world of broken bolts was not enough to explain how Martha's blog had defied the odds. Logically it shouldn't have happened. There were too many hurdles in the way and at any point the bubble could have been burst. We would not have fought it if it had happened and as long as we drifted down to earth gently we wouldn't have been upset. The London Olympics seemed to have reinvigorated the country with a new willingness to applaud its champions for their achievements and Martha seemed caught up in the new spirit. We'd made no attempt to plan or plot the course we took expecting, and some days hoping, that the world would move on without us. The fact it hadn't was testament to the emotional power the blog had.

Written without agenda but with the heart and passion that nine year olds give their work, NeverSeconds had the capacity to enthral readers and encourage them. Strength to me was a description of the weight a bolt could carry not the power a bunch of words had to change the world. There was no other word for it though and the strength the blog had was powerful enough to bring children and adults together, initially to debate school dinners and then onward to helping those with less. The kids in Lirangwe were so exuberant in their thanks for the help of the Friends of NeverSeconds that we had all been

taken aback. The huge praise was a reflection of the massive difference it made to their lives. It was saddening to think that more children in Malawi don't receive a Mary's Meals than do. There was more to be done and we could only hope that sharing the visit would motivate more people to support Mary's Meals in any way they could.

Our media commitments weren't yet over. On return to the UK Martha and I were due to visit the BBC One Show sofa to help promote the documentary. Dates had changed and instead of a few days recovery we were now expected to be on the day after we landed back from Malawi. Nerves about flights home were swapped for nerves about live television. Martha was keen to go but worried she'd make a mistake.

"Don't worry. They won't ask you anything you haven't been asked before," I encouraged her.

"But they'll ask me about why I started the blog again. I've told people that so many times already."

"It's a new audience though. Some may never have heard of NeverSeconds or Mary's Meals."

"I'll tell them but it's the last time," she said firmly. Martha was ready to move on and I understood her reluctance to keep looking backwards. It was nearly six months ago now and to her that was an age.

"You've enjoyed it though?"

"Yes, it's been awesome. I never knew I could write so much or help so many kids until I tried."

"What about the future? The presenters may ask you what's next."

"That's easy," she said, skipping to the door. "Being ten and playing more netball."

Acknowledgements

To Rebecca, Joe and Polly for putting up with us writing. Agogos John, Jane, Barry and Anne for picking up the phone, listening and farm sitting. Our family for their support, wise words and counsel. Richard and Catalina for a great party that sewed a seed. The Friends of NeverSeconds for saving the blog and donating. Hazel, Steve and Cliff for slowing down on our runs so I could keep up. Jamie Oliver for his kindness and support. Mr Maddox for inspiring a girl to write and Mrs Stankey for permission to blog. Kim and all the staff at Mary's Meals in Scotland and Malawi for offering so much assistance. The Charity Children and their families who supported kids helping others. Nick Nairn for his backing, encouragement and the hours of post ban interviews. Ray, Laura, Chris, Steve and Gillian for going above and beyond to help get the message out from Malawi. The children of Malawi for sharing with us. Dee, Nancy, Colin, George and Fergus for their farming friendships. Our guest bloggers, Blodwyn, NAH and NAYK, CJ, Pavlova, Enzo Buzz and Giorgio Bros, Camp Director FireFly and the Wanderers, The Hungry Birds, Hansik, Jagej, Doni and JAM for bringing their stamp to the blog. Wiktor for introducing us to Malawi in all its forms and his staff at Fisherman's Rest, Blantyre, for looking after us. UWC Atlantic College and the Extra Mural centre for helping Rebecca and I see the world in a different way. Helen and Mark from Cargo for doing their very best to make the book a success and for maximising meals to Malawi.